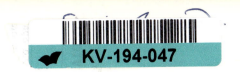

DO IT YOURSELF REVISION FOR NURSES
Book 5

DO IT YOURSELF REVISION FOR NURSES

BOOK 5

E. J. Hull B.A., S.R.N., R.N.T.

Formerly Principal Tutor, Luton and Dunstable Hospital

and

B. J. Isaacs S.R.N., Part 1 C.M.B., R.N.T.

Principal Nursing Officer (Training)
Luton and Hitchin Hospital Management Committee

Examiner for the General Nursing Council
for England and Wales

Baillière Tindall · London

First published 1972

© 1972 Baillière Tindall
7 & 8 Henrietta Street, London, WC2 8QE
A division of Crowell Collier and Macmillan Publishers Ltd.
ISBN 0 7020 0410 3

Published in the United States of America
by the Williams & Wilkins Company, Baltimore

Reprinted 1972

Reproduced and printed by photolithography and bound in
Great Britain at The Pitman Press, Bath

PREFACE

Encouraged by the kind reception given to the first four books in this series, we have prepared two further books. As before, these are based on questions, mostly from recent State Final Examination papers, with 'model answers'. We hope, however, that they are radically different from the usual kind of 'model answer book', because they embody ideas about learning which we have tried out on many student nurses, and which have proved to be popular and successful. They are not intended merely to prepare students for examinations, but also to encourage them to study intelligently.

The 1969 Syllabus of the General Nursing Council lays down that 'the study of any condition from which a patient may be suffering either of a general or specialised character should include:

Applied anatomy and physiology
Cause
Symptoms and well-known signs
Reasons for investigation
Treatment
Nursing care to include observations and records
Normal course of the disease
Complications
Social aspects and rehabilitation.'

This has been borne in mind in the choice of questions; and as far as possible each one deals with several of the above aspects of a condition.

Books 5 and 6 complete our series. They include some chapters on more specialized aspects of nursing, as well as further questions of a general nature, and we hope that students will find them a useful addition to their bookshelves

Each chapter has three parts: a list of *points to revise,* the *question,* and the *model answer,* with a scheme for marking. The method of using it is explained in more detail in the introduction *To the student.*

The aims of the books are:

1. To reduce to a minimum the number of errors made when the student answers the question. Students do not learn anything from answering questions badly. Thus the *points to revise* pages set out in some detail just what the student should revise before attempting the question. This has the additional advantage of giving her something definite to look up, so that she does not waste her time by revising too much too vaguely.

2. To cause the student to respond as soon as possible to each point which she has revised. This explains why the 'points to revise' are limited to those which are actually to be used in her answer. It is only when a student has responded to, or used, what she has heard or read that she really learns it.

3. To give the student immediate knowledge of her results. Because of tutor shortage, students' varying off-duty between study blocks, and so on, we have all had the experience of correcting questions which cannot be returned to students for several days. By then, they have often lost their first interest, and tend not to notice corrections. In this method, on the other hand, the student corrects and marks her own answers at once by the *model answers*. This consolidates her knowledge of what she has done well, and prevents erroneous ideas from becoming fixed.

In view of some comments which we have received on Books 1 and 2, we would point out that these books are *not* meant to be used as textbooks or reference books. The answers only provide a guide to be used by the nurse in correcting her own work *done under examination conditions*. Thus, for example, we have omitted the *doses* of drugs, as in practice doses must always be checked by the prescription; and it is impossible to remember the dose of every drug which you might mention in a question.

Our acknowledgements go to many past and present student nurses in this hospital, who have helped us by their cooperation and enthusiasm.

E.J.H.
B.J.I.
January 1972   Luton and Dunstable Hospital

CONTENTS

Page

Introduction
To the student — how to use this book   1

Accident Work (including First Aid)
1   Burns   3
2   Accidents and their prevention   9
3   Sudden collapse   15
4   First aid and later treatment   21
5   Organization of a Casualty Department   27

Ward Teaching (3)
6   Questions about teaching theory   33
7   Insulin reaction   41
8   Acute rheumatism   47

Female Reproductive System (2)
9   The menstrual cycle. Amenorrhoea   53
10 Ruptured ectopic gestation   59
11 Hysterectomy   65
12 Senile vaginitis   71

Disturbances of Metabolism
13 Obesity   77
14 Hypothermia   83
15 Oedema   89

Alimentary Tract (2)
16 Difficulty in swallowing   95
17 Haematemesis   101
18 Perforated peptic ulcer   107

Urinary System (2)

19	Carcinoma of kidney. Nephrectomy	113
20	Renal colic	119
21	Acute renal failure	125

22	**Radiotherapy**	131

INTRODUCTION

TO THE STUDENT – HOW TO USE THIS BOOK

'Do It Yourself Revision' is intended for busy student nurses, who want to revise, but perhaps do not quite know where to start. Success in studying depends on doing a little, often; so we suggest that you start early, and not just before your examinations. But please note that the purpose of the book is *revision*; so you should start with those chapters which deal with subjects about which you have *already learnt.*

Each chapter starts with a list of *points to revise.* This includes different aspects of a subject, which you ought to study in order to answer the question in the next section. Depending on how much time you have to spare, this revision can be spread over some days. We suggest that you might try to cover one chapter each week.

When you have finished revising (but not before), turn over the page and write the answer to the question you will find there. You should do this as if you were in the examination room, allowing yourself not more than 35 minutes.

When you have written your answer (not before), you turn over to the the next page. Here is a *model answer*, with a scheme of marking. You correct and mark your own work, if possible immediately after doing the question.

The most important part of each chapter is the *points to revise*. These points do not only enable you to answer one particular question once set in a State Final Examination. If you use them carefully they give you the background knowledge and understanding of the subject, which should help you in answering *other* questions which the examiners may think up about it. More important, you will really learn something. So resist the temptation to skim over the revision pages and rush on to the question and answer. One way of doing this is to get together in a small group to do the revision, and sometimes, even, to write a "group" answer. You can learn a lot by discussing with one another; and the brilliance of your "group" might astonish you.

The advantages of marking your own work are; firstly, that you know your results immediately, while the subject is fresh in your mind, and sooner than if you gave it to a tutor to mark. Secondly, you take more notice of corrections if you make them yourself. Thirdly, you can do your revision at any time you find convenient. Lastly, if you get bad marks, nobody will know except yourself.

The answers are sometimes given in note form. This does not mean that you should write them in this way; but it may make it easier for you to pick out the points as you correct it.

Bearing in mind that in the State Examination you have only 30 to 35 minutes in which to plan and write an answer, our model answers do not contain every bit of information which you might possibly include. We have put in the main points which we, as examiners, would expect to be included in a limited time. Under examination conditions, one hardly ever writes a perfect answer. So do not be discouraged; if you get 70% you are doing quite well.

Keep a record of your marks for each question. You will find that they improve as you get more practice in writing answers. If you do get poor marks for a question, you will learn quite a lot as you correct your answer. You can prove this if you try the same question again after a few weeks.

The way you arrange your *time* in examinations is of vital importance. Not much is said about this in these books, but your tutor will give you guidance. In addition we recommend a very useful article entitled "Against the Clock" by E. Robbins, which appeared in the *Nursing Times* of 27th July, 1972.

ACCIDENT WORK (INCLUDING FIRST AID)
1. Burns

Points to revise

1. List the dangers and complications of severe burns.

2. Make some notes on:
   (a) Treatment given to counteract these dangers during the first three days in hospital
   (b) Methods which you have seen used for the local treatment of extensive burns

3. List the important points in the nursing care of a patient with severe burns. Include your observations and the records which you would keep.

4. Make some notes on:
   (a) The psychological difficulties which may be encountered by a small child who has to be admitted to hospital.
   (b) The problems affecting the family of a child who has to have prolonged treatment in hospital

When you have revised these points, and not before, turn over the page.

Question

Without consulting any book, write the answer to the question on this page. You should not take more than 35 minutes to plan and write your answer.

A 3-year-old girl is brought to the Casualty Department with severe burns on the trunk. Discuss:

(a)	Her immediate care	25%
(b)	The problems associated with the admission to hospital of a child of this age	25%
(c)	Her nursing care while in hospital	25%
(d)	The advice you would give her parents when the child is discharged	25%

When you have finished your answer, turn over and correct it by the 'model answer' overleaf.

Model answer

(a) *Immediate care* (25 marks)

When the child is admitted, the mother must be reassured as far as possible, and asked to stay with the child to comfort it (3 marks). The little girl will be given an analgesic such as nepenthe or morphine (2 marks).

The first essential is to replace the fluid which is being lost from her burns (2 marks). Clothing is cut off (1 mark), and the doctor estimates the proportion of body surface affected (2 marks). From this he calculates the amount of fluid needed to replace what is being lost (2 marks) and to supply normal intake (1 mark).

An intravenous infusion of plasma will be started immediately (4 marks). Instruments for venesection may be needed for this (2 marks). The amount to be given over each three hours will be prescribed, and must be strictly adhered to (2 marks).

The child will be catheterized, so that the amount of urine passed can be measured every hour (3 marks). This shows whether enough fluid is being given (1 mark).

(b) *Problems associated with admission* (25 marks)

A child of this age is extremely dependent upon her mother, and separation when she is very ill must be avoided if possible (3 marks). Accommodation for the mother must be found in hospital so that she can stay with the child (3 marks). This means that the mother will have to make arrangements for the care of her family at home (4 marks), which may involve the Medical Social Worker and the Public Health Authority (3 marks). The father may need persuasion to allow his wife to remain with the child (2 marks).

The mother will probably feel guilty, and will be very distressed, so she will need support and encouragement (4 marks); she may need sedation at first (1 mark).

Another problem is that this child is too young to understand the reasons for treatment, and will probably be very fretful; so nurses and the mother will need great patience (5 marks).

(c) *Nursing care* (25 marks)

Burns of the trunk are usually exposed, as it is difficult to keep dressings in position (2 marks). Therefore, to avoid cross-infection, the child should be admitted to a cubicle or side-ward (2 marks), and great care must be taken to prevent raising dust when it is cleaned (1 mark). Masks and gowns must be worn by nurses when they are in the cubicle (1 mark), and hands must be washed before doing anything for the child (1 mark). The mother must be taught to take the same precautions (1 mark). The temperature of the cubicle must be kept between 21° and 26°C (70° and 80° F).

The child will be put into a cot so that if possible she is not lying on the burnt surfaces (1 mark), i.e. in a prone position if the burns are on the back, or lying on her back if they are on the front of the trunk (1 mark). She should lie on sterile pads which are changed when they become wet (1 mark).

Until the surfaces of the burns have coagulated, the intravenous infusion of plasma will be continued, and it is essential to make sure that the prescribed amount of fluid runs in (1 mark). The catheter will be released hourly at first (1 mark); and if the hourly output is less than 15 ml it should be reported (1 mark).

Intake and output of fluid will be recorded until the danger of fluid loss is past (1 mark). The temperature, pulse and respiration are taken and charted 4-hourly (1 mark).

As soon as she can take them, the child will be given fluids by mouth (1 mark). She will need a high-protein diet (3 marks). The mother is encouraged to help in washing and feeding her (1 mark), and in keeping her amused (1 mark).

When the burns are beginning to heal, the child can be given a daily bath, to which salt or an antiseptic such as Savlon has been added (1 mark). This helps to keep the areas clean (1 mark), and also helps her to move about (1 mark).

(d) *Advice to parents* (25 marks)

If the child has areas of full-thickness burns, she may have to return to hospital for skin-grafting later; and arrangements for this should be discussed fully with her parents (5 marks).

They should be advised to give her a good diet, with plenty of milk, meat and eggs (3 marks), as she may be anaemic as a result of her burns (1 mark). If she has to take iron medicine or vitamin supplements, the importance of these should be explained (1 mark).

The mother will be advised to keep the child's skin clean by giving her a daily bath (1 mark); and she should also understand if the doctor wants any treatment to the skin, such as applying cream or olive oil to keep it supple (3 marks). The clothing should be light — preferably of

cotton (2 marks) — and should be changed frequently (1 mark).
The parents should be advised to let their daughter live as normal a life as possible, and not to spoil her or make an invalid of her (3 marks). If her mother has not stayed with her in hospital, they should be warned that she may be difficult to manage and make great demands on her mother, and that they will need patience to overcome this (5 marks).

ACCIDENT WORK (INCLUDING FIRST AID)
2. Accidents and their Prevention

Points to revise

1. List the dangers which may be incurred by young children from the following:
   - (a) Toys
   - (b) Kitchen equipment
   - (c) Poisonous substances

2. List ways in which young children may sustain:
   - (a) Burn and scalds
   - (b) Injury due to falls
   - (c) Asphyxia

3. Make notes on the ways in which you, as a young mother (or father), could safeguard your child from the above dangers.

4. Make notes on:
   - (a) The first aid treatment which should be given for a child who has inhaled a foreign body
   - (b) The immediate treatment of this child in hospital

When you have revised these points, and not before, turn over the page.

Question

Without consulting any book, write the answer to the question on this page. You should not take more than 35 minutes to plan and write your answer.

(a)	What accidents may befall children in the home?	20%
(b)	How may they be avoided?	50%
(c)	What would be done for a child who had inhaled a 2p piece?	30%

When you have finished your answer, turn over and correct it by the 'model answer' overleaf.

Model answer

(a)   *Accidents to children in the home* (20 marks)

Accidents which may occur are:

Burns from any kind of open fire, which may set clothing alight
(2 marks). Children may also clutch at the bars of an electric fire
(1 mark) or may play with matches (1 mark). They can knock over
oil-stoves while playing (1 mark).

Scalds from pulling saucepans or kettles over themselves (1 mark) or
from falling into buckets or washing machines containing hot water
(1 mark).

Poisoning from drinking poisonous cleaning materials (1 mark), from
taking tablets which look like sweets (2 marks) or from eating poisonous
seeds and berries from the garden (1 mark).

Asphyxia from putting plastic bags over their heads (2 marks), turning
on gas taps (1 mark) or inhaling foreign bodies (1 mark).

Crushed fingers from playing with machines such as mangles, mincers or
folding chairs (2 marks).

Cuts from playing with knives and scissors (1 mark).

Fractures, bruises and abrasions from falling downstairs, out of windows
or off swings (2 marks).

(b)   *Avoiding accidents* (50 marks)

Children should never be left alone in the house (3 marks).
Young children should not be left alone in a room where there are
dangers such as mechanical appliances (2 marks), fires (2 marks) or oil-
stoves (2 marks). Oil-stoves should not be put where they can be
knocked over or in a draught (1 mark). All fires should have secure
guards (3 marks).
Children's clothing should be non-inflammable (3 marks), and they
should wear pyjamas rather than nightdresses (1 mark).
Saucepans on stoves should have their handles turned away from the
room (2 marks). Kettles and teapots should not be left near the edge
of a table (2 marks).

Anything which is dangerous must be kept out of reach of small
children at all times (1 mark); for example, matches (1 mark), scissors
and knives (1 mark), plastic bags (1 mark) and cleaning fluids (1 mark).
Medicines and tablets should be locked in a cupboard out of reach

(3 marks). No poisonous fluids should be put into lemonade or milk bottles (1 mark).

A play-pen helps to keep a small child safe (2 marks). He should have toys to distract him from playing with dangerous things (2 marks). For example, he can have toy scissors to prevent him from wanting to play with dangerous ones (1 mark). Toys for small children should be large, and not have small detachable parts which they can put in their mouths (3 marks). They should be guaranteed as safe from other dangers, such as poisonous lead paint (1 mark).

Upper floor windows should have bars fixed (2 marks); and there should be a gate at the top of the stairs while children are young (2 marks). It may help a busy mother if she can take the child to a play group on some days (1 mark), or send him to a nursery school (1 mark). As soon as they are old enough to understand, children should be taught to avoid dangers (2 marks). For example, they can be taught not to eat poisonous berries in the garden (1 mark). When they are older, they should be shown how to use such things as matches and scissors safely (2 marks).

(c) *Treatment for a child who has inhaled a 2p piece* (30 marks)

The child should immediately be held upside down and slapped on the back, in an effort to make him cough out the 2p piece (8 marks) If this is not successful, he should be reassured (1 mark), and put in the semi-prone position (3 marks). He must be taken to hospital immediately by car, or if there is no car, an ambulance should be sent for urgently (4 marks). If he becomes blue, he can again be held upside down (1 mark). Nothing should be given by mouth (3 marks).

In hospital, the child's neck and chest will be X-rayed in order to find the position of the foreign body (2 marks). The doctor will then pass a laryngoscope (1 mark) or a bronchoscope (1 mark) under general anaesthetic (1 mark), and the coin will be removed (1 mark).

The child may be kept in hospital for 24 hours in case oedema of the larynx occurs (2 marks). In the case of a small child arrangements will be made for the mother to stay with him (2 marks).

Points to revise

1. List the causes of unconsciousness.

2. Make a list of the priorities in the first aid treatment of an unconscious patient.

3. Make sure you could describe the steps which should be taken in a case of cardiac arrest.

4. Make some notes on the responsibilities of nurses when an unconscious patient is admitted, with regard to:
    (a) Treatment of the patient
    (b) Care of his belongings
    (c) Dealing with his relatives

When you have revised these points, and not before, turn over the page.

Question

Without consulting any book, write the answer to the question on this page. You should not take more than 35 minutes to plan and write your answer.

A middle-aged man collapses unconscious in front of you in the street.

(a) What immediate steps would you take to deal with
     the situation?   40%

(b) Enumerate the possible causes of sudden
     unconsciousness.   20%

(c) What are the special responsibilities of the nursing
     staff in the Casualty Department when an unconscious
     patient arrives at the hospital?   40%

Hint to students: Notice that part (b) only carries 20% of the marks. Remember to *enumerate* only; do not waste time explaining the causes of unconsciousness in detail.

When you have finished your answer, turn over and correct it by the 'model answer' overleaf.

Model answer

(a)   *Immediate steps to be taken* (40 marks)

I would look to see if the man was breathing (2 marks). If he is not, and has no pulse, he should be laid on his back, with a rolled-up coat under his shoulders to extend his neck (5 marks). He will then need artificial respiration by the mouth-to-mouth (*or* mouth-to-nose) method (3 marks and external cardiac massage (3 marks). As this needs two people, I would ask any by-standers whether they could help me (2 marks). The more experienced person should give the massage, while the other gives artificial respiration (3 marks). Another by-stander should be sent to telephone for an ambulance (1 mark) by dialling 999 (1 mark), or to find a policeman who will do this (1 mark).

If the man is breathing, his collar should be loosened (1 mark), and he should be turned into the semi-prone position (3 marks). His dentures and spectacles should be removed (2 marks). Someone should be asked to summon an ambulance or fetch a policeman (1 mark).

I would then look in the man's pockets to see if he was carrying a card (*or* I would look for a disc worn round his neck or wrist) stating that he was a diabetic (2 marks), an epileptic (2 marks) or taking cortico-steroids (2 marks). If he was a diabetic he might be carrying sugar, and a lump could be put on his tongue to dissolve if he were not too deeply unconscious (2 marks).

I would remain with the patient until the ambulance arrived (2 marks), and hand over to the ambulance personnel, telling them what I had done and anything I had found out (2 marks).

(b)   *Causes of sudden unconsciousness* (20 marks)

1.   Massive myocardial infarction (3 marks).
2.   Cerebral haemorrhage (2 marks).
3.   Cerebral thrombosis (1 mark).
4.   Severe subarachnoid haemorrhage (2 marks).

If you have put 'stroke' or 'cerebrovascular accident' instead of items 2, 3 or 4, count 3 marks.

5.   Epileptic fit (2 marks).
6.   Acute alcoholism (2 marks).
7.   Insulin reaction (3 marks).
8.   Fainting (2 marks).
9.   Sub-dural haemorrhage following head injury (3 marks).

(c)   *Responsibilities of nursing staff in Casualty Department* (40 marks)

The first responsibility of the nursing staff is to make sure that the patient is breathing (4 marks). If artificial respiration and cardiac massage have been started, they must continue this until medical help is available (1 mark).

An unconscious patient who is breathing must be put in the semi-prone position (2 marks), and suction should be applied if necessary to keep his airway clear (2 marks). A mouthgag and artificial airway should be at hand (3 marks).

The nursing staff are also responsible for seeing that the doctor is informed of the patient's arrival (2 marks). If relatives are with the patient, they should be reassured that the doctor is coming and will see them when he has examined the patient (2 marks).

If the patient is unaccompanied, any information about his identity should be obtained from the ambulance personnel or policeman who are with him (2 marks). The police should be asked to contact relatives and bring them to the hospital (3 marks).

The patient's pulse should be taken (2 marks). His temperature and blood pressure will be taken once he is undressed (1 mark). Two nurses should undress him carefully, ready for the doctor's examination (2 marks). If his name is known, an identity bracelet must be attached to his wrist or ankle (3 marks).

The nurses should count and check any money or other valuables, and list these in the property book (2 marks). They must see that the valuables are locked up by the appropriate department according to the rules of the hospital (2 marks). The patient's clothing can be given to his relatives, or else listed and put away later (2 marks). Staff of the Casualty Department must see that dentures and spectacles accompany the patient to the ward (2 marks).

As soon as possible the ward to which the patient is to be admitted should be notified (1 mark). The patient must not be left unattended, as the Casualty Department is responsible for his care and safety until he reaches the ward (2 marks).

ACCIDENT WORK (INCLUDING FIRST AID)
4. First Aid and Later Treatment

Points to revise

1. Revise the general principles involved in first aid treatment.

2. Make notes on the particular dangers connected with:
    (a) Head wounds
    (b) Fractures of the lower limb
    (c) Wounds contaminated by soil
    (d) Chemical burns of eyes

3. Make notes on the principles of treating the above injuries:
    (a) Immediately
    (b) Later

4. List any special points to remember in dealing with emergencies involving:
    (a) Children
    (b) Elderly people

When you have revised these points, and not before, turn over the page.

Question

Without consulting any book, write the answer to the question on this page. You should not take more than 35 minutes to plan and write your answer.

Describe the first-aid measures and subsequent treatment that may be required in the following situations:

(a)	Profuse bleeding from the scalp following a road traffic accident.	25%
(b)	An elderly lady who has fallen down stairs at home and fractured a femur.	25%
(c)	A farmer who has sustained a penetrating wound of a foot.	25%
(d)	A child who has accidentally spilled caustic soda in her eyes.	25%

When you have finished your answer, turn over and correct it by the 'model answer' overleaf.

Model answer

(a) *Profuse bleeding from the scalp* (25 marks)

First aid. Provided that the patient is conscious, sit him up and support him (2 marks).

Apply a large (2 marks), clean dressing, such as a small towel or folded handkerchiefs (2 marks), and secure with an improvized bandage (1 mark). Reassure the patient that he will soon get treatment in hospital (1 mark). Keep him covered with coats or rugs (1 mark).

Transport the patient to hospital by car or ambulance (1 mark).

Later. In hospital the patient will be examined by a doctor (1 mark). His skull will be X-rayed (1 mark).

Hair will be cut and shaved from round the wound (2 marks). The wound will be cleaned and sutured under a local anaesthetic (2 marks). A long-acting antibiotic will be ordered and given by intramuscular injection (1 mark). A course of tetanus toxoid injections will be started if the patient has not previously been immunized; if he has had a course within 5 years, a booster dose will be given (2 marks).

The patient will be admitted to hospital for at least 24 hours, in case there is underlying brain damage (2 marks). During this time observations will be made on his pulse (1 mark), blood pressure (1 mark), pupil reactions (1 mark) and level of consciousness (1 mark).

(b) *Elderly lady with fractured femur* (25 marks)

First aid. The patient should be comforted and the first-aider should explain that she will have to go to hospital (2 marks).

She should be covered with a blanket or rug (1 mark) and can have a pillow put under her head (1 mark). She should not be given any food or drink (1 mark).

The injured leg should be gently straightened and tied to the other leg with a towel or scarf placed round the thighs and knees with another around the lower leg (3 marks).

If there is a telephone nearby, the patient's own doctor may be notified (1 mark); if not, an ambulance should be sent for (1 mark). A relative or friend should accompany the patient to hospital, if possible (1 mark).

Later. In hospital the patient will be undressed and examined by a doctor for other injuries (2 marks). An X-ray will be taken (1 mark). An analgesic such as pethidine (or other suitable example) will be ordered and given by injection (2 marks). She will be admitted for immediate operation for internal fixation of the fracture by means of a

24

Smith-Petersen nail, McLoughlin's pin and plate or Austin-Moore's prosthesis (3 marks for any of these three methods). A blood transfusion will be given (2 marks). If surgery has to be postponed, the leg will be temporarily immobilized in Russell traction (3 marks).
After operation, early mobilization and rehabilitation will be carried out (1 mark).

(c) *Penetrating wound of foot* (25 marks)

First aid. If possible, the wound should be cleaned with an antiseptic (2 marks) before being covered with a clean dressing or handkerchief, which is bandaged on or secured with strapping (3 marks).
The patient should be taken to hospital (1 mark).
Later. In the Casualty Department, the foot is thoroughly cleaned (2 marks) and the wound excised to eliminate deep infection under a local or general anaesthetic (4 marks). It is then sutured (1 mark).
A long-acting antibiotic will be ordered and given (*or* you may have given an example such as benzathine penicillin or Penidural) (2 marks).
Tetanus toxoid will be given (2 marks): either the first injection of a course of three (1 mark), or a booster dose if the patient has already been immunized (1 mark). If the course is started, a card is given to the patient with particulars and the date of the next injection (1 mark).
The farmer will be admitted, or sent home to rest his foot if he has someone at home to look after him (3 marks). He will be seen in the Casualty Department, or by his own doctor, in 3 days time (2 marks).

(d) *Caustic soda burns of eyes* (25 marks)

First aid. The eyes should be immediately washed out with cold water (5 marks).
The child should be comforted and reassured (2 marks); the mother must also be calmed and allowed to nurse the child on her lap (2 marks).
If available, castor oil drops can be put into the eyes (2 marks), and both eyes should be covered with improvized pads and a bandage (2 marks). Child and mother should be taken to hospital by car or ambulance (1 mark).
Later. The child is admitted and the mother allowed to stay (2 marks).
The eyes are examined (1 mark) and atropine drops instilled (2 marks).
An antibiotic ointment such as chloramphenicol (*or* other example) is put into the eyes (2 marks), and they are covered with pads and a bandage (1 mark).
Scarring may necessitate corneal grafting to restore vision (3 marks).

ACCIDENT WORK (INCLUDING FIRST AID)
5. Organization of a Casualty Department

We are assuming that this chapter will be used chiefly by students who have worked in a casualty department or accident service. You would probably get more out of the 'points to revise' if you discussed them with another student who also had this experience.

Points to revise

1. Make some notes on the help which the Sister or Charge Nurse in charge of a Casualty Department should be able to give:
   (a) To her senior nursing staff
   (b) To her student nurses

2. List the different areas or sections which you found in the department in which you worked.

3. Good relationships with other departments can help in the service given to the patients in the casualty department. With what departments may the nurse in charge have to communicate:
   (a) In order that patients are not kept waiting in the department unnecessarily?
   (b) In order that the staff have all the equipment which they need in order to cope with the work?

4. In what circumstances may the nurse in charge have to communicate with the police?

When you have revised these points, and not before, turn over the page.

Question

Without consulting any book, write the answer to the question on this page. You should not take more than 35 minutes to plan and write your answer.

Discuss the responsibilities of a senior nurse in the organization of a Casualty Department.   100%

When you have finished your answer, turn over and correct it by the 'model answer' overleaf.

Model answer

N.B. As this is an essay question, each of you will have answered it in a different order and in different words; so you may have to look through the model answer carefully in order to find the points which you have included.

We have allocated the marks in the following proportions:
   Responsibilities of the senior nurse for her own nursing staff and students — 40 marks.
   Her responsibilities in running the department, including communications with other departments inside the hospital — 50 marks.
   Her responsibilities in communicating with people outside the hospital — 10 marks.

As this question is about organization and management, it does not include the individual nurse's duties towards patients.

Responsibilities of a senior nurse in the organization of a casualty department (100 marks)

The nurse in charge has the responsibility of allocating the nursing staff within the department (5 marks). This will include delegation of responsibility to her senior nursing staff for different areas (5 marks), such as the accident theatre, fracture clinic, major and minor injuries sides (2 marks for any two examples). She must make sure that these people know their particular responsibilities (5 marks), and should be able to advise them about their work (3 marks).

She must make the best use of different grades of staff according to their abilities (3 marks); this involves using part-time staff to the best advantage (1 mark). She must inform the nursing administration of her staffing needs (2 marks), and report absences of staff (2 marks). The senior nurse is also responsible for making sure that student nurses get the experience they need (5 marks). Each student should spend some time in each area of the department (2 marks). She should go through their records of practical instruction with the student nurses, and fill them in herself (4 marks). She will have to give reports to the Matron (*or* the nursing administrator) on students and other grades of staff (1 mark).

She must make sure that the department is properly equipped so that it can run smoothly (5 marks). This will include ordering new equipment

(2 marks) and making sure that the necessary orders for replacements of equipment and drugs (4 marks) are sent in regularly at the correct times (2 marks). She must see that her staff report to her on losses (2 marks), and on repairs which are necessary (2 marks), and make sure that these are dealt with (2 marks). She must also see that there is a sufficient supply of clean linen (2 marks) and that the department is kept clean (2 marks).

These duties make it necessary for her to have good communications with with other departments inside the hospital (3 marks): the Central Sterile Supply Department (2 marks), the Pharmacy (2 marks) and the Domestic Superintendent (2 marks). She will have to consult the Hospital Secretary's department (2 marks) on portering services (1 mark), maintenance (1 mark) and care of patients' property (1 mark). Other departments with which she must be in contact are the X-ray department (2 marks) and the Laboratory, which supplies blood (2 marks). She must work in co-operation with clerical staff who deal with appointments (2 marks), and with the Medical Director's office (2 marks), so that she knows where beds are available (2 marks). She must also know which teams of medical staff are on call at different times for emergencies (3 marks).

The senior nurse in charge is also largely responsible for communications between the department and various people and agencies outside the hospital (2 marks). She has to know about informing the coronor and police if a patient is brought in dead or dies in the department (2 marks), informing the police about accidents (1 mark) and about requesting them to contact relatives (1 mark). She has to arrange for ambulances and other transport when patients are transferred (2 marks). She may need to be in contact with factory health services (2 marks).

WARD TEACHING (3)
6. Questions about Teaching Theory

In many final papers, part of a question asks 'What would you teach junior nurses about . . . ?', or 'How would you explain this to a junior nurse?'. The mistake often made in answering these questions is to make the answer sound like a page from a textbook. This only shows what *you* know about the subject; it is not a complete answer to a question about *teaching.*

Question 1

Here is an example of this kind of question.

A patient aged 40 years with mitral incompetence has been admitted to hospital with heart failure.

(a)	Describe the treatment and nursing care of this patient.	50%
(b)	What observations would you make while this patient is in hospital?	25%
(c)	*What would you teach the junior nurses about this condition?*	25%

Below are two answers to (c). Choose the one you think is the better, and list reasons *why* you think it better.

(i) I would tell the junior nurses that the mitral valve, between the left atrium and ventricle of the heart, normally prevents blood from returning from the ventricle to the atrium. Mitral incompetence means that the valve will not close properly, so the atrium has difficulty in emptying, which causes it to become enlarged. Eventually this leads to back pressure on the pulmonary veins and lungs. The lungs become congested, causing breathlessness, which is the first sign of heart failure. This increases as the condition progresses; and sometimes sudden attacks of dyspnoea occur, called cardiac asthma. The condition is usually caused by rheumatic fever during childhood.

(ii) I would ask one of the nurses to draw a diagram of the heart, showing the valves and the blood vessels by which blood enters and leaves. I would ask them the function of the valves, and explain that mitral incompetence means that the mitral valve will not close properly, so that blood flows back through the valve. Using the diagram, I would show how there is a 'build-up' of blood in the left atrium, leading by degrees to back pressure in the pulmonary veins and lungs. An X-ray of the patient's chest could be used to show that his atrium was enlarged. I would ask the nurses what symptoms they had noticed in this patient, and lead them to account for his breathlessness or for attacks of cardiac asthma. I would ask if they knew what disease often caused damage to the heart; we could look in his notes to see if he had a history of rheumatic fever.

When you have written reasons for your choice, turn over.

You were meant to choose (ii) as the better answer.

Both answers contained almost exactly the same information; but (i) was just 'textbook', while (ii) had some ideas about how to teach.

The main points to notice are:

1. Answer (i) did not mention the *patient*, who was the reason for this bit of teaching, at all. Answer (ii) used the patient, his X-ray and his case notes in order to make the teaching interesting and *real*. It is the great advantage of ward teaching that you have real patients, not imaginary ones, on the ward. Also, most nurses are much more interested in patients whom they know than in descriptions of diseases in textbooks. Because of this patient, these junior nurses might be much readier to learn and remember about mitral incompetence than they will be in a few months' time when they are in a study block. That is why it is important to give them explanations *on the ward.*

2. Answer (i) only mentioned the 'junior nurses' once, and then continued as if they were not there. It *told* them everything, and telling people things is not the only, or the best, way of teaching. The junior nurses should be brought into the discussion and made to take some part in it.
   Answer (ii) brought the students in by asking them to draw a diagram and answer questions. They were treated as intelligent people, who already knew something about the heart, and who could think and use their powers of observation.

3. Answer (ii) built on what the junior nurses already knew. It did not, however, take this for granted, but questioned them about it before proceeding to new material. In any kind of teaching, you always try to proceed from what is already known; so you must make sure that it *is* known.

4. Answer (ii) made use of a diagram; this makes explanation of the consequences of mitral incompetence a good deal easier to follow.

On the opposite page there is another question for you to consider.

Here is another question with a section on teaching junior nurses.

Question 2

A 20-year-old student is admitted to hospital with bronchial asthma.

(a)	*How would you explain this condition to junior nurses?*	20%
(b)	In an acute breathless attack what action would you take and what treatment is given?	50%
(c)	Describe the care and treatment of this patient after discharge from hospital.	30%

Consider your answer to (a), and make some notes on:

1.   The facts you would expect the junior nurses to know already, and how you would test this knowledge.

2.   The facts which you hope to teach them, arranged in a logical order.

3.   Ways in which you could base your teaching on the patient mentioned in the question.

When you have made your notes, and not before, turn over the page.

1. *Facts which you would expect junior nurses to know*

You can always assume that junior student nurses have some elementary knowledge of anatomy and physiology, although they are only given an outline of this in the Introductory Course. Here, you could assume that they should know what is meant by 'bronchi' and 'bronchioles'; and that they should know that the bronchioles open into air-spaces (*or* air-sacs) in the lungs. They should also know that there is an interchange of oxygen and carbon dioxide between the air-spaces and blood vessels in the lungs. You could test this knowledge by asking them to draw diagrams of the bronchial tree and of the air-sacs in the lung.

2. *Facts which you hope to teach*

In asthma the smaller bronchi and bronchioles go into spasm (*or* become constricted), especially when the patient is trying to breathe out. Therefore there is a wheezing sound during expiration.

Asthma is usually an allergic condition; that is, the patient is sensitive, generally to something which he inhales, such as dust or pollen, which does not affect other people. Contact with this is always liable to start an attack of asthma. In people subject to it, attacks are often brought on by mental or physical stress, or by infection.

3. *Ways in which you could base teaching on the patient*

You can draw the junior nurses' attention to the way the patient is breathing during an attack, and ask them whether it is during inspiration or expiration that there seems to be more difficulty. You can also draw attention to his wheezing. From this you would go on to explain what is happening to his bronchi and bronchioles.

You could ask the nurses what they notice about the patient's colour, and explain that he is cyanosed because he retains expired air in his lungs and is not getting enough oxygen.

His case notes can be used to go into his history. They will show that he has had previous attacks of asthma. Old notes may show that the causes have been investigated, e.g. by skin tests, and may reveal that he is sensitive to some particular thing, such as feathers or cats. This leads to explaining that asthma is an allergic condition. His notes will also show if he is a student, and he could be asked when he takes his examinations, as worry about them might explain his recent attacks; this could be pointed out to the nurses. Or his notes might show that he had been suffering from chest infection, or that he was sensitive to penicillin. These could then be explained as possible causes of asthmatic attacks.

Now continue with the next question on the page opposite.

Here is the last question in this chapter.

Question 3

A patient is admitted to hospital with carcinoma of the stomach.

(a)	Describe the relations of the stomach to other structures.	20%
(b)	List the functions of the normal stomach.	20%
(c)	*How would you explain to a junior nurse how this disease causes the patient's symptoms?*	20%
(d)	Describe the special postoperative nursing care following gastrectomy.	40%

Consider your answer to (c), and make notes as before on:

1. The facts you would expect the junior nurse to know already, and how you would test this knowledge.

2. The facts which you hope to teach them, arranged in a logical order.

3. Ways in which you could base your teaching on the patient mentioned in the question.

When you have made your notes, and not before, turn over the page.

1. Facts you would expect the junior nurse to know

You could expect her to know something of the anatomy of the stomach: its shape, and that it is part of the alimentary tract between the oesophagus and duodenum; and that food remains in it for up to 4 hours, and then passes out through the pyloric sphincter. Probably the best way of testing this would be to ask her to draw a diagram and label the parts. You could also ask her what she knew about gastric juice, and could expect her to know that it is normally acid. If she had seen nasogastric tubes aspirated, you could expect her to have noticed that the gastric juice was tested with litmus paper.

2. Facts which you hope to teach

You would probably need to start by explaining simply what 'carcinoma' is; i.e. that it is an abnormal growth of cells, which multiply very rapidly: what lay people call 'cancer'.

The patient loses weight, and may be very wasted and anaemic. This is because the carcinoma grows rapidly, and uses up the nourishment which should be supplied to normal tissues. It is like a parasite, growing at the expense of the patient, who is practically starving.

He will also suffer from loss of appetite and indigestion. For normal gastric digestion, gastric juice must be acid; and the acid also promotes appetite. Carcinoma of the stomach results in a lack of acid in gastric juice, which explains these symptoms.

If the growth is large and near the pylorus, it may cause a pyloric obstruction. This results in vomiting.

3. Ways in which you could base teaching on the patient

If the patient looked ill and wasted, you could ask the junior nurse what she noticed about his appearance; she would have noticed that he is very thin and pale, and that his skin is dry and inelastic. This would lead you to explain how the carcinoma uses up much of his available nourishment.

If a barium meal X-ray had been done, you could show the growth or malignant ulcer on this.

You could ask the patient in front of the nurse about his symptoms of indigestion and loss of appetite; or use his case notes, in which these symptoms will be recorded.

If a nasogastric tube had been passed, you could show the nurse that the gastric juice did not contain acid by aspirating it and testing it with litmus paper.

WARD TEACHING (3)
7. Insulin Reaction

As this chapter contains another question on ward teaching, you should have worked through chapter 6 before you start on it. Below are other points to look up if necessary.

Points to revise

1. List signs and symptoms which may occur with an insulin reaction.

2. List the steps you would take if you suspected that a patient was about to have such a reaction.

3. Make notes on what you would teach a diabetic patient about his insulin.

When you have revised these points, and not before, turn over the page.

Question

Without consulting any book, write the answer to the question on this page. You should not take more than 35 minutes to plan and write your answer.

A diabetic patient had 40 units of soluble insulin at 8 a.m. At 8.20 a.m. he becomes restless and aggressive and is sweating profusely.

(a)	What would you do in this situation?	10%
(b)	How could similar attacks be prevented in future?	30%
(c)	How would you explain this attack to the junior nurses in the ward?	60%

When you have finished your answer, turn over and correct it by the 'model answer' overleaf.

Model answer

(a) *Dealing with the patient with insulin reaction* (10 marks)

As quickly as possible the patient should be given some sugar or glucose dissolved in water (5 marks), or anything else easily available, such as a sweet fruit drink or glass of milk (1 mark for any suggestion). He should be tactfully persuaded to sit down and take it (1 mark). As soon as he recovers, he should be given his breakfast without delay (1 mark). The reaction should be reported to the doctor, so that any necessary adjustments of his insulin dose or diet can be made (2 marks).

(b) *Prevention of future attacks* (30 marks)

In future, care should be taken that this patient does not have to wait too long for a meal after being given his insulin (3 marks). The reason for the attack should be explained to him (2 marks), and he should be given some sugar lumps to keep in his locker, so that he can take one if he feels another similar attack coming on (2 marks). He will now know the warning signs; and should also be advised to carry some sugar in his pocket after his discharge from hospital (2 marks). The doctor will have to decide whether his dose of insulin needs reducing (1 mark) or his diet increasing (1 mark). The nurses must test his urine and record the results regularly (2 marks), and a complete absence of sugar in it should be pointed out to the doctor, as it is a warning that his insulin or diet may need adjusting (3 marks). The patient will be taught to test his own urine, and should also know this (3 marks). It is also important to impress upon the patient that he must eat the prescribed amount of carbohydrate in his diet, otherwise he will be likely to get an insulin reaction (5 marks). Before he leaves hospital he should know that, if he is ill, other carbohydrate foods can be replaced by taking sugar or glucose (2 marks): 1 lump of sugar or 1 teaspoonful of sugar or glucose for every 5 units of insulin (2 marks). He should also know that he may have a reaction if he takes more exercise than usual, so that he is prepared at such times to take some sugar (2 marks).

(c) *Explanation to the junior nurses* (60 marks)

I should expect the junior nurses to know that the patient was a diabetic and that he was being given insulin, so I would ask them his diagnosis (2 marks) and what drug he was being given (2 marks) and

why (2 marks). They would probably know that diabetics cannot make insulin for themselves (4 marks), and that insulin enables people to metabolize (*or* use) sugar (4 marks). I would ask them about these points, and if they did not know would explain them (1 mark).
I would then say that the insulin a diabetic is given must be exactly enough to balance the carbohydrate in his diet (4 marks). If he has too little insulin, he will have a high blood sugar — too much sugar in his blood; but if he has too much, his blood sugar will be too low (4 marks). This patient had too little sugar in his blood (5 marks); and this affected his brain, causing the signs and behaviour which they saw (5 marks). I would find out if they had noticed him perspiring (2 marks), and point out that this is a usual sign of insulin reaction (2 marks), and indicates the need to give the patient sugar at once (2 marks). I would point out how quickly he recovered when given sugar (5 marks).

I would say that soluble insulin starts to act rapidly, within about 15 minutes (5 marks), and they might then suggest if asked that the reason for the attack was that the patient has been given insulin but had not yet had breakfast (5 marks). I could then stress that after soluble insulin patients should be given a meal as soon as possible (3 marks). I would also explain how important it was for a patient taking insulin to eat all the carbohydrate foods in his diet at each meal, to avoid disturbing the balance between the insulin and the carbo-hydrate (3 marks).

WARD TEACHING
8. Acute Rheumatism

Points to revise

1. List the special points about the ways nursing sick children differ from nursing sick adults.

2. Make sure you know how acute rheumatism occurs, and how the disease presents.

3. Make sure you could name the complications which can be caused by acute rheumatism, and the steps taken to try and prevent them.

4. List (a) the drugs and (b) the investigations used in this disease.

5. List the points you would mention to the child's mother, and the advice you would give her:
   (a) While her son is in your ward with acute rheumatism
   (b) When he is discharged

When you have revised these points, and not before, turn over the page.

Question

Without consulting any book, write the answer to the question on this page. You should not take more than 35 minutes to plan and write your answer.

You are in charge of a children's ward. A child aged 7 years has been admitted suffering from acute rheumatism.

(a)	Describe the nursing care he will require.	40%
(b)	Describe the treatment.	30%
(c)	What would you teach the student nurses about this child's condition and nursing care?	30%

When you have finished your answer, turn over and correct it by the 'model answer' overleaf.

Model answer

(a) *Nursing care* (40 marks)

The nurse in charge of the ward should introduce herself to the child, and try and gain his confidence (1 mark). She should explain that she wants him to stay quietly in bed and remain lying down so he will get better quickly (2 marks). The mother will probably be with him and should be allowed to stay until he has settled down in the ward (1 mark).

The little boy should be made as comfortable as possible in bed with only one soft pillow (1 mark). A bed-cradle is put in to keep the bed-clothes away from his painful joints (1 mark); a flannelette sheet is put under the cradle for warmth (1 mark). If his joints are very painful, they can be wrapped in warmed wool, or gamgee, and lightly bandaged for comfort (2 marks).

As he will be pyrexial, a 4-hourly temperature chart is commenced (2 marks). Recordings on a sleeping pulse chart may also be requested as this gives a truer reading when a child is not excited (2 marks).

The patient will need bathing, in bed, once or twice a day, as he is likely to perspire a good deal at first (2 marks). Pyjamas and bed linen will need to be changed frequently for the same reason (1 mark). Finger- and toe-nails will be kept clean and short (1 mark) and his hair kept tidy by brushing and combing (1 mark). If he is neglected, or unclean when admitted, his hair should be inspected for parasites and disinfested if necessary (1 mark).

During bathing and bedmaking, everything should be done for the child and he should be lifted to avoid rolling him onto his painful joints (2 marks). He should be lifted on and off bedpans also (1 mark).

The mother is encouraged to visit frequently (1 mark) and should be allowed to help with her son's personal toilet. She can help him to clean his teeth after meals and before he settles for the night (2 marks), and she can feed him and amuse him (2 marks). The nurse must explain to the mother that the child must not get excited (1 mark); suitable amusements are being read to, watching television and listening to the radio (2 marks for any 2 suggestions).

Plenty of fluids should be given and these can be taken through a drinking-straw; favourite drinks should be given (2 marks). He will probably only want to eat ice-cream and light puddings at first, but his diet should be increased as soon as he feels better (1 mark).

As the pulse and erythrocyte sedimentation rates settle, the child can be given extra pillows and gradually allowed to sit up and do more for himself (2 marks). He can be given books and toys to play with, as long as he keeps quiet (1 mark for suitable amusement).

Mobilization must be gradual, and even when the child is allowed up he should not get too boisterous with the other children (1 mark). Any rise in pulse is a sign that he is too active and a further period of rest may be ordered (2 marks). Convalescence should be long (1 mark).

(b) *Treatment* (30 marks)

Salicylates in the form of soluble aspirin (*or* Disprin) 300 mg will be ordered 4-hourly for 5—7 days (3 marks). This brings down the temperature (1 mark) and stops the pain (1 mark).

Penicillin will be ordered for 48 hours to be given intramuscularly (2 marks). After this it will be given orally for 2—3 weeks, and then continued in smaller daily doses for several years (*or* until the child leaves school) to prevent further throat infections (3 marks). Corticosteroids (*or* prednisolone, betamethazone or other example) will be ordered if there is no response to the other drugs after 48 hours, or if there are abnormal heart sounds when the child is admitted (2 marks). These drugs help to prevent damage, or further damage, to the heart (2 marks). They will probably be given for a week in decreasing doses (1 mark).

On admission a throat swab is taken for bacteriological examination. It will be repeated after 7—10 days to see if the antibiotics are having effect (2 marks).

The haemoglobin estimation will show if the child is anaemic and if so, iron will be ordered (1 mark).

Blood will be taken each week for erythrocyte sedimentation rate and a chart will be kept of the results (1 mark).

The mother must be instructed about further treatment when the child leaves hospital: that he must have plenty of protein foods and an adequate vitamin intake (2 marks), that he should have frequent periods of rest during the day (1 mark) and should not go back to school until instructed by the doctor (1 mark). The child must not play active games for at least a year (1 mark).

If home conditions are poor, it may be necessary to send the child to a residential school for a time and one must be found where his health can be watched, his drugs given and supervised resting periods allowed (3 marks). The medical social worker may help to get the family rehoused, as dampness and overcrowding are predisposing factors in this disease (2 marks).

An appointment for the child's first out-patient attendance should be given the mother when she takes him from the ward (1 mark).

(c) *Teaching student nurses about acute rheumatism* (30 marks)

They can be told that the disease starts with a throat infection (1 mark) and should be asked if they know which micro-organisms cause this (1 mark).

It is explained that the haemolytic *Streptococcus* produces toxins (2 marks). They should be able to say what antibiotic the child is having; if not, they can be referred to the drug sheet and told why this is the drug being given (1 mark).

The nurses can then be asked if they know why the child is being nursed at complete rest (3 marks) and a short explanation can be given about the effects on the heart (2 marks); they may know the names of the coats of the heart, so that endocarditis and myocarditis can be discussed (2 marks). They can look at the temperature and sleeping pulse charts and be asked why they are being recorded so often (2 marks); they may be able to suggest why tachycardia is present (1 mark), why the sleeping pulse is of importance (1 mark) and why the temperature is returning to normal (1 mark). If the junior nurses cannot answer these questions, they should be given adequate explanation in simple terms (1 mark).

The nurses can be asked to describe the child's pains; if they cannot do so, the little boy can tell them. The typical 'flitting' pains can be pointed out and the nursing care to prevent further discomfort when making his bed and bathing him (2 marks). They should be able to say what drug stops the pain (1 mark).

They may not realize how aspirin causes sweating so the need for baths, changing of linen can be pointed out (2 marks).

The junior nurses may be able to suggest how to keep the child happy, and the sort of amusements which are suitable while he is lying flat (1 mark). As they are working on a children's ward, they may have ideas about free visiting and why it is a good thing to allow the mothers to help with their children's care (2 marks).

If the child is still being given penicillin intramuscularly, the senior nurse should go with one of the juniors pointing out why it is necessary to tell the child: 'It *will* hurt a little, but will soon be over if you keep still' rather than 'It won't hurt'. This is also a good opportunity to stress the importance of two nurses always being there when giving injections to a child, asking them why this is so (2 marks).

If the E.S.R. is measured on the ward, the junior nurses can be asked what this is, and how they read the result. If they have not seen the equipment, they can be shown (2 marks).

FEMALE REPRODUCTIVE SYSTEM (2)
9. The Menstrual Cycle. Amenorrhoea.

Points to revise

1. Make sure you know the meanings of the following terms:

    Amenorrhoea
    Puberty
    Menopause

2. 'Amenorrhoea' is said to be (a) primary or (b) secondary. Make sure you know the difference between these two kinds, and make lists of the causes of each.

3. List the ways in which disorders of menstruation may be investigated.

4. Revise the menstrual cycle and make sure you could account for the parts played by:
    (a)   The pituitary gland
    (b)   The ovaries
    (c)   The endometrium

You may find it helpful to make a chart like the one below, and fill it in as you revise to illustrate the changes which occur during the cycle.

Days	1	14		26	28
Pituitary					
Ovaries					
Endometrium					

When you have revised these points, and not before, turn over the page.

Without consulting any book, write the answer to the question on this page. You should not take more than 35 minutes to plan and write your answer.

(a)	Give an account of the causes of amenorrhoea.	40%
(b)	What investigations may be carried out to determine the causes of amenorrhoea?	20%
(c)	Describe the physiological control of the menstrual cycle and the cyclical changes in the body which occur.	40%

When you have finished your answer, turn over and correct it by the 'model answer' overleaf.

Model answer

(a)   *Causes of amenorrhoea* (40 marks)

Absence of menstrual periods may be *primary* (2 marks) when the patient has never menstruated (1 mark), or *secondary* (2 marks) which occurs after the periods have started (1 mark).

Primary amenorrhoea may be normal (*or* physiological) before puberty (2 marks), or abnormal (*or* pathological) after the age of 17 (2 marks). This may be due to pituitary gland malfunction (1 mark) or absence (1 mark) or malfunction of the ovaries (1 mark). The uterus may be absent (2 marks) or underdeveloped (*or* infantile) (2 marks). Another cause is haematocolpos (2 marks) where there is malformation of the vagina; the menstrual flow is prevented from escaping by a membrane lying across the vagina (2 marks). The blood collects and causes enlargement of the vagina and uterus (1 mark). Treatment is by incision under an anaesthetic (1 mark).

Secondary amenorrhoea is normal during pregnancy (2 marks) and lactation (1 mark); and after the menopause (2 marks). It is abnormal in some constitutional diseases such as tuberculosis, renal or liver diseases, anaemia, pituitary and other endocrine disorders, malabsorption conditions or acute infections (4 marks for any 4 examples). Hormone disturbances which occur around puberty (2 marks) and the menopause (2 marks) may cause episodes of amenorrhoea. Other causes are psychiatric illnesses due to stress such as homesickness, bereavement, change of job, desire for or fear of pregnancy (4 for any 4 examples).

(b)   *Investigations* (20 marks)

A careful history is taken by the doctor (1 mark). The patient is given a complete physical examination (2 marks) and her urine is tested for abnormalities (2 marks). A chest X-ray is taken to exclude tuberculosis (1 mark).

An internal pelvic (*or* vaginal) examination is performed (2 marks). It may be necessary to examine the patient under a general anaesthetic (2 marks) when a diagnostic dilatation and curettage may also be performed so that the endometrium can be examined histologically (4 marks).

The patient may be asked to take and record her temperature on waking, each day for 3 months to find out whether or not ovulation is occurring (3 marks).

Blood tests will be done (1 mark) such as haemoglobin estimation

(1 mark), white cell count and erythrocyte sedimentation rate (1 mark for either).

(c)   *The menstrual cycle* (40 marks)
This is controlled by hormones from the pituitary gland (1 mark) and the ovaries (1 mark). Each cycle lasts approximately 28 days (1 mark), from the start of one menstrual period to the start of the next (1 mark). About the second day of the menstrual period (1 mark), the pituitary gland starts to secrete follicle stimulating hormone (*or* F.S.H.) (2 marks). This causes one primitive follicle (1 mark) on the surface of one of the ovaries (1 mark) to begin enlarging (1 mark). The ovum inside the follicle ripens (1 mark) and the follicle fills with fluid; this is known as the Graafian follicle (2 marks). It produces the hormone oestrogen. As the amount of oestrogen in the blood increases (1 mark), the endometrium starts to regenerate (*or* thicken) (2 marks) and after 2 or 3 days, menstruation ceases (2 marks).
Ripening of the ovum and enlargement of the Graafian follicle continue until about day 14 (1 mark) when the follicle ruptures (1 mark) and the ovum escapes into the peritoneal cavity (1 mark). This is called ovulation (1 mark).
In the second half of the cycle, the pituitary gland produces luteinizing hormone (*or* L.H.) (2 marks). This causes the space on the ovary, left after ovulation, to fill with a yellow substance called the corpus luteum (2 marks). The corpus luteum produces two hormones: oestrogen (1 mark) and progesterone (2 marks).
Oestrogen and progesterone cause further thickening of the endometrium (2 marks) to prepare it for a possible pregnancy (1 mark). Its blood supply increases, its glands enlarge and extra glycogen is laid down (2 marks for any 2 changes).
After a further 12 days (1 mark) if conception does not take place (*or* if no pregnancy occurs), the corpus luteum disintegrates (1 mark), the supply of hormones stops (1 mark) and the endometrium shortly afterwards breaks down and bleeds: menstruation starts (1 mark).

FEMALE REPRODUCTIVE SYSTEM (2)
10. Ruptured Ectopic Gestation

Points to revise

1. Make sure you understand the term 'ectopic gestation'.

2. List the signs and symptoms of internal (or concealed) haemorrhages and the reasons why these occur.

3. Revise the structure and function of the Fallopian tubes.

4. List the *essential* points in dealing with surgical emergencies:
    (a)   During the admission of the patient
    (b)   When preparing the patient for theatre

When you have revised these points, and not before, turn over the page.

Without consulting any book, write the answer to the question on this page. You should not take more than 35 minutes to plan and write your answer.

A young married woman is admitted in a collapsed state with a ruptured ectopic gestation.

(a)	Describe the normal anatomy and physiology of the Fallopian tube.	20%
(b)	Why does a ruptured ectopic gestation give rise to such a collapsed state?	20%
(c)	What are the priorities in the admission procedure?	30%
(d)	How would you prepare the patient for theatre?	30%

When you have finished your answer, turn over and correct it by the 'model answer' overleaf.

Model answer

(a) *Anatomy and physiology of the Fallopian tube* (20 marks)

Each Fallopian tube is about 10 cm (4½ in) long (1 mark) and leads from the upper part of the uterine cavity (1 mark) in a backwards direction (1 mark).

The tube is narrow and hollow, the lumen being continuous with the uterine cavity (2 marks). It is curved (1 mark), and the end widens out with finger-like projections (*or* is fringed or fimbriated) (2 marks). The tube has thin muscular walls (1 mark) and is lined with ciliated epithelium (3 marks).

Under the end of the tube lies an ovary (1 mark), which is attached to one of the fimbriae (1 mark). The tube is covered by a fold of peritoneum called the broad ligament (2 marks).

Function. After ovulation, the fimbriae direct the escaped ovum into the lumen of the tube (2 marks). The cilia waft the ovum along the tube into the uterine cavity (2 marks).

N.B. If you have drawn a diagram which shows the shape and position of the tube, like the one below, *substitute 5 marks* for the second sentence above.

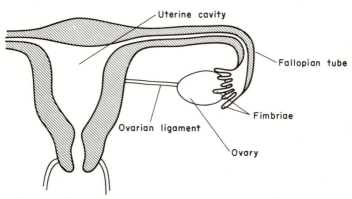

(b) *Reasons for patient's collapsed state* (20 marks)

During early pregnancy the blood supply to the reproductive organs increases (1 mark).

The uterine artery, a branch of the aorta, passes very near to the walls of the Fallopian tube, and as the tube ruptures there will be an internal haemorrhage into the peritoneal cavity (5 marks). This causes a sudden fall in blood pressure (4 marks). The severe pain caused by irritation of the peritoneum adds to the patient's collapsed state (3 marks).

The patient looks very pale because blood supply to the periphery is very poor (2 marks) and her skin will feel cold and clammy (2 marks). She may feel faint because of cerebral anoxia (1 mark).

Fear adds to the shock (1 mark), and the ambulance journey, or the time-lag, may have made her condition deteriorate (1 mark).

(c)   *Priorities in admission procedure* (30 marks)

Because the patient is shocked and in pain, she will need very gentle lifting and handling with as little moving as possible (3 marks). The foot of the bed (or trolley) can be elevated (2 marks).

As soon as the doctor has made his diagnosis, he will order an analgesic such as morphine or papaveretum (Omnopon) (*or* other suitable example) which the nurse should give as soon as possible (5 marks).

The patient should be reassured and told that she will have to have an operation, but that she will make a good recovery (2 marks).

If she is unaccompanied, her husband should be sent for (2 marks).

As the patient is a young married woman, there may be social problems such as young children at home, or older children coming from school, and the medical social worker can be asked to help in these matters (4 marks).

An intravenous infusion will be set up; probably normal saline or a plasma substitute will be used first, while arrangements are made for grouping and cross-matching of blood for transfusion (5 marks).

The operating theatre should be informed as this is a surgical emergency (1 mark).

The patient's particulars are taken from here if she is fit enough; if not, most of these can wait until her husband arrives (2 marks).

Her clothing and other property is listed, and money and valuables listed, checked and locked away for safe-keeping (3 marks).

She may be taken to the ward, or be sent straight to theatre from the Casualty (*or* Accident) Department (1 mark).

(d)   *Preparing the patient for theatre* (30 marks)

Nurses must work quickly but calmly to prevent alarming the patient (2 marks). Undressing, all treatment and movement of the patient must be as gentle and smooth as possible (3 marks).

A consent for operation form must be filled in and signed by the patient and/or her husband and an explanation should be given about the procedure involved (4 marks).

A specimen of urine should be obtained and tested for abnormalities, and the results written in the patient's notes. If this is not possible, the doctor should be told as catheterization may be required (5 marks).

The abdomen, vulva and perineum should be shaved (3 marks).

The nurse should make sure that the skin of the abdomen is clean, particularly the umbilicus (3 marks). If there is vaginal bleeding, the vulval area should be swabbed with antiseptic and a sterile sanitary pad applied (2 marks).

The patient is dressed in operation gown (1 mark), socks (1 mark) and cap (1 mark). An identity bracelet is filled in and attached to her wrist or ankle (2 marks). Prostheses and jewellery are removed (1 mark). Premedication, such as atropine or scopolomine, is given as ordered (2 marks).

FEMALE REPRODUCTIVE SYSTEM (2)
11. Hysterectomy

Points to revise

1. Make sure you can draw a diagram of the uterus, labelling its main parts.

2. Make sure you could give an account of the structure of the uterus.

3. List the structures which lie near the uterus.

4. List the *specific* points in the nursing care needed by a patient undergoing major gynaecological surgery:
    (a) Before operation
    (b) After operation

5. List the complications which may occur after abdominal hysterectomy.

When you have revised these points, and not before, turn over the page.

Without consulting any book, write the answer to the question below.
You should not take more than 35 minutes to plan and write your
answer.

Describe the uterus and list the important anatomical relations.   30%

A patient of 35 is admitted to hospital for hysterectomy.
(a)	Describe her preoperative preparation.	30%
(b)	Describe the postoperative nursing care.	30%
(c)	What common complications may follow this operation?	10%

Hint to students: As the question states 'hysterectomy', and as the
patient is only 35 years old, the authors have taken this question to
mean *ABDOMINAL hysterectomy* and have worded the 'model answer'
accordingly.

*When you have finished your answer, turn over and correct it by the
'model answer' overleaf.*

Model answer

The uterus and its anatomical relations (30 marks)

The uterus is a hollow (1 mark), pear-shaped (1 mark) organ, which lies in the pelvis (1 mark). Its walls are made of thick (*or* 3 layers of) involuntary muscle tissue (1 mark) called the myometrium (1 mark), well supplied with blood vessels (1 mark), and able to stretch during pregnancy (1 mark). The lining is called endometrium (1 mark) and is controlled by hormones which cause cyclical changes (3 marks). The lining of the cervical canal is of mucous membrane (1 mark).

The part above the uterine cavity is called the fundus (1 mark), the part containing the cavity the body (1 mark) and the lower, narrow part the cervix (1 mark).

The cavity is continuous with the lumen of the Fallopian tubes (2 marks), and with the cervical canal below (1 mark). The internal os is at the upper end of the cervical canal (1 mark), and the external os opens into the vagina (1 mark).

N.B. If you have drawn a diagram, showing the shape of the uterus, and labelled as below, substitute 9 marks for those in the description.

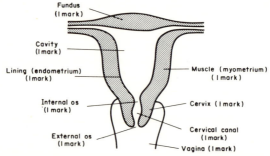

Important anatomical relations are: bladder and urethra (1 mark), ureters (1 mark), Fallopian tubes and ovaries (1 mark), vagina (1 mark), peritoneum and pouch of Douglas (1 mark), broad ligament (1 mark), rectum (1 mark), perineal body (*or* levatores ani muscles) and supporting ligaments (2 marks) and the ovarian and uterine arteries and veins (1 mark).

(a) Preoperative preparation (30 marks)

The patient is sent for 24–48 hours before her operation (1 mark). She should be greeted by name and reassured (1 mark). Her particulars are taken (1 mark) and the nurse checks that the patient and her husband have signed the consent form (1 mark), and answers any queries they may have (1 mark). The patient is shown her bed and the ward lay-out and is asked to get undressed (1 mark). She should be in bed, as the doctor will give her a full physical examination (2 marks).

A specimen of urine is saved and tested, and the results are charted in the notes (2 marks). A mid-stream specimen of urine (1 mark) and a high vaginal swab are sent to the laboratory for bacteriological examination and microscopy (1 mark).

The patient should not smoke (1 mark). The physiotherapist will teach her breathing and leg exercises, so that she will know what to do after her operation (1 mark).

Her abdomen, pubic area and perineum are shaved (2 marks), and the patient has a bath (1 mark). The evening before operation the bowel is emptied by means of suppositories or an enema (2 marks). A hypnotic is usually ordered by the doctor to ensure a good night's sleep (1 mark). On the day of operation, the patient has another bath and is *either* shown how to use the bidet *or* has the vulval area swabbed (1 mark for either). A sterile pad is secured with a T-bandage (1 mark). No food or drink is given for 4 hours before operation (1 mark). The patient is asked to empty her bladder (1 mark) and puts on an operation gown, socks and cap (1 mark). Hair-grips, prostheses and jewellery are removed and nail-varnish taken off (1 mark). Her wedding ring may be covered with adhesive tape (1 mark). She must again be reassured (1 mark). An hour before she goes to theatre her premedication is given and she is left to sleep (2 marks).

(b)   *Postoperative nursing care* (30 marks)

Until the patient regains consciousness, a nurse stays with her to ensure that here airway is clear (1 mark); her head should be kept to one side, or she should be in the semiprone position (1 mark). The nurse records her pulse and blood pressure every half hour until they are satisfactory (2 marks); later they are taken hourly, then 4-hourly (1 mark). Once she is conscious and her condition satisfactory, the patient has her face and hands washed (1 mark), and her own nightdress put on (1 mark), and and is gradually sat up (1 mark). She is encouraged to practise her breathing and leg exercises (1 mark), and shown how to support her wound while coughing (1 mark).

The wound and sanitary pad should be inspected frequently for excess bleeding, the wound being repacked and the pad changed when necessary (2 marks).

As soon as necessary the postoperative analgesic is given, and will probably need repeating 4- or 6-hourly for the first 48 hours (2 marks). If an intravenous infusion is in progress it should be maintained according to instructions, probably for 24 hours (1 mark). A fluid balance chart is kept for 3 or 4 days (1 mark). If there is no vomiting, sips of water can be given, and later free fluids (1 mark).

Special care must be taken to see that the patient passes urine, and it may be necessary to catheterize her if no urine is passed after 12 hours; this depends on the surgeon's wishes (2 marks).

The patient may have abdominal discomfort for the first 48 hours. This may be relieved by passing a flatus tube (*or* giving carminatives) (1 mark for either). She should be reassured that the discomfort will pass off once she starts eating, has a bowel action and becomes mobile (1 mark). The day after operation, most patients are well enough to sit out of bed; and on subsequent days the patient begins to get up and walk about (1 mark). While in bed, she is helped to care for her teeth and hair and given a daily bed bath (1 mark). Until she can use the bidet, the vulval area is swabbed with antiseptic and fresh sterile pads are applied, vaginal loss being noted and reported to the doctor if excessive (1 mark). Diet is gradually increased to one with adequate protein and vitamin C to aid healing (1 mark). A mild laxative, suppositories or small enema is given on the third day is necessary (1 mark). The wound is inspected, but dressings are not disturbed unnecessarily. Clips and/or sutures are removed after 5–10 days (2 marks).

The patient can probably leave hospital 10 days after the operation, but should be advised to go away for a period of convalescence (1 mark). Before she leaves an appointment is made for her to attend Out-patient Department in 3 months' time (1 mark).

(c) *Common complications* (10 marks)
Reactionary haemorrhage may occur during the first 24 hours (1 mark), and secondary haemorrhage, due to infection, after 7–10 days (1 mark). Shock may occur during the immediate postoperative period (1 mark). In the first 24 hours there may be retention of urine (2 marks). Infection may arise in the chest (1 mark), urinary tract (1 mark) or wound (1 mark).

Deep venous thrombosis may occur after 5–7 days (1 mark); pulmonary embolism after 7–10 days (1 mark).

FEMALE REPRODUCTIVE SYSTEM (2)
12. Senile Vaginitis

Points to revise

1. Make sure you could describe the structure of the vagina.

2. Make sure you know what changes occur in the vagina:
    (a) Before puberty
    (b) During reproductive life
    (c) After the menopause

3. List the signs and symptoms which may occur in senile vaginitis.

4. List the micro-organisms which may infect the vagina after the menopause.

5. Make sure you know how the above condition is investigated and treated.

6. List the points you would stress when advising a patient with senile vaginitis how to prevent further infection.

When you have revised these points, and not before, turn over the page.

Question

Without consulting any book, write the answer to the question on this page, You should not take more than 35 minutes to plan and write your answer.

An elderly woman attends the Out-patient Department with senile vaginitis.

(a)	Explain with reference to anatomy and physiology how this condition occurs.	50%
(b)	What treatment and advice may be given?	50%

When you have finished your answer, turn over and correct it by the 'model answer' overleaf.

Model answer

(a) *How senile vaginitis occurs* (50 marks)

The vagina is lined with stratified epithelium (*or* skin) (3 marks). Friction between the two walls is prevented by mucus (2 marks) made in glands of the cervix, which protrudes into the upper part of the vagina (3 marks). The lining is thick and rich in glycogen during the reproductive years (2 marks), but thinner and lacking in glycogen after the menopause (2 marks). The blood supply to the vagina also decreases after the menopause (1 mark).

Senile vaginitis is a localized vaginal infection which occurs after the menopause (5 marks). It is usually caused by the *Escherichia coli* (*or Bacillus coli*) (3 marks) but can be caused by *Streptococcus faecalis, Monilia albicans* (*or* thrush) or *Trichomonas* (2 marks for any 2).

After the menopause, the natural resistance to infection in the vagina is lowered (2 marks). During reproductive life, oestrogen (3 marks) maintains the thick vaginal lining and Doderlein's bacilli (3 marks), normal vaginal commensals (*or* non-pathogenic bacteria), act on the glycogen and produce lactic acid (3 marks). This acts as a natural antiseptic (2 marks). Once the supply of oestrogen ceases, the acidity is no longer present (3 marks).

Because of the inflammation, there will be profuse offensive discharge which may be purulent or blood-stained (3 marks).

Because the bladder and urethra are adjacent to the vagina, there may be frequency of micturition (3 marks).

There may also be discomfort in the pelvis and dyspareunia (2 marks). The condition is common in diabetics (3 marks).

(b) *Treatment and advice* (50 marks)

In the Out-patient Department the patient's urine is tested to exclude diabetes (3 marks).

A thorough physical examination is done by the doctor (2 marks); an internal pelvic examination is done to exclude malignant disease of the cervix or uterine body (3 marks). The vagina is examined under direct vision and swabs are taken from any ulcerated areas for bacteriological culture (5 marks). During examination, any other causes for the discharge may be discovered, such as a neglected foreign body (*or* a supportive pessary) or a uterine prolapse (2 marks for either).

Treatment of senile vaginitis is based on restoring the acidity, thus increasing its resistance to infection (5 marks). This may be done by the administration of oestrogens by mouth for 2—3 weeks, or in the form of pessaries which the patient is taught to insert into the vagina each night (5 marks).

Oestrogen pessaries may be combined with lactic acid to increase the acidity further (3 marks). The patient may be able to give herself vaginal douches of lactic acid 0.5% (or 2 teaspoonsful of vinegar in 500 ml water) daily (3 marks). Another method of employing oestrogens is in the form of vaginal cream, such as dienoestrol (or other example), applied by means of a special applicator into the top of the vagina (3 marks).

As this condition is very distressing to the patient, she will need a great deal of reassurance that it will get better with treatment (2 marks). She should be advised to pay particular attention to personal hygiene by washing the vulval area and careful drying twice a day (3 marks). Underwear should be changed and washed daily (2 marks) and knickers are better made of cotton than nylon or wool which may increase the vulval irritation (2 marks).

If the patient lives on her own, she may need advice about her diet as she is less likely to cook well-balanced meals for herself (1 mark). She should be warned that there may be slight vaginal bleeding when she stops the oestrogen tablets, or pessaries, and if this occurs she should go to her doctor or return to the clinic (2 marks).

If any other disease or infection was discovered at examination, such as diabetes or a specific infection, this is treated (or you may have said that antibiotics or chemotherapeutic agents are given for other vaginal infections) (3 marks).

The patient should be seen again in the out-patient Department in 4 weeks' time (1 mark).

DISTURBANCES OF METABOLISM
13. Obesity

Points to revise

1. List causes of obesity.

2. List any medical reasons why patients are advised to lose weight.

3. Make notes on the advice you would give to a fat person about:
   (a) Her diet
   (b) Her general way of life
   (c) Any other help she might be able to obtain in reducing her weight

   Make sure you could give reasons for offering this advice.

When you have revised these points, and not before, turn over the page.

Question

Without consulting any book, write the answer to the question on this page. You should not take more than 35 minutes to plan and write your answer.

(a) What are the causes, dangers and complications of obesity?   50%

(b) Describe in detail a reducing diet. What other treatment may be given?   50%

When you have finished your answer, turn over and correct it by the 'model answer' overleaf.

Model answer

(a) *Causes, dangers and complications of obesity* (50 marks)

The commonest cause is over-eating (4 marks). Often this is a habit which starts early in life, so that a fat baby or child becomes a fat adolescent and adult (1 mark). Sometimes unhappiness is a contributing cause, an individual finding comfort in eating (2 marks).

Bad eating habits may also be responsible: that is, eating too many sweet and starchy foods (3 marks). These habits may be due to ignorance of nutrition (1 mark), or to buying cheap, filling foods because more expensive foods, such as protein foods and fruit, cannot be afforded (1 mark). Beer-drinking is also a cause of obesity (1 mark).

Lack of exercise and a sedentary occupation may also be partly responsible for obesity (2 marks).

It is a condition which tends to run in families (1 mark). This probably partly because the children tend to over-eat like their parents (1 mark), but also partly because differences in the rate of metabolizing food are hereditary (1 mark).

Patients with myxoedema put on weight because they metabolize food very slowly (3 marks). Others may gain weight when treated with anti-thyroid drugs or following thyroidectomy (1 mark).

A pituitary deficiency may be responsible for fatness, causing the 'fat boy' type of child (1 mark). Prolonged treatment with corticosteroids can also lead to obesity (1 mark); and endocrine changes at puberty or the menopause sometimes contribute to it (1 mark).

Obesity often leads to hypertension (3 marks), which in turn may lead to strain on the heart (*or* left-sided heart failure) (2 marks) and other complications such as strokes (2 marks).

It also makes patients more likely to suffer from coronary thrombosis (3 marks); and in any kind of heart disease, the added weight puts extra strain on the heart (3 marks).

Obese patients are also more liable to severe chest infections, and more likely to die from them (2 marks). They run a greater risk if they have to undergo surgery for this reason (1 mark), and are also more likely to develop deep venous thrombosis (1 mark).

Obesity in middle-aged women is often associated with diabetes developing at that time (3 marks).

Fat adolescents may have psychological difficulties, being over-sensitive, shy and depressed (3 marks). They may try to slim without medical supervision, and this can be dangerous (1 mark); or even go to extremes and develop anorexia nervosa (1 mark).

(b) *Reducing diet and other treatment for obesity* (50 marks)

A reducing diet must have a low calorie value (2 marks), usually 1000 to 1200 calories per day (2 marks). As this diet does not meet the patient's needs for energy and heat, she loses weight because she is forced to metabolize her own body fat (2 marks).

The intake of carbohydrate foods must be greatly reduced (2 marks). The patient must give up sugar and sweets (1 mark) and foods such as jam and cakes which contain sugar, including foods such as tinned fruit and fruit juices which contain it (2 marks for any 3 correct examples). If necessary saccharin can be substituted for sugar (1 mark), and the patient may have special 'diabetic' jams, chocolate, tinned fruit or fruit juices which contain no sugar (2 for any 2 correct examples).

Starchy foods, such as bread and potatoes are allowed in limited quantities (2 marks). Fat is also limited (2 marks), and generally given as a ration of butter (2 marks). Foods cooked in fat are avoided (2 marks). Milk, which contains both fat and some sugar, is generally limited to about half a pint a day (1 mark).

The patient may have plenty of protein foods (3 marks), such as lean meat, white fish (not fried), hard cheese and eggs (2 marks for any two examples). Protein speeds up the rate of metabolism and therefore helps in slimming (2 marks).

To satisfy the appetite, quite a lot of green vegetables and salads should be provided in the diet (3 marks); but no salad cream or oil (1 mark). Fruit is also allowed (2 marks), except for some kinds which contain a good deal of sugar, such as dates, grapes and bananas (1 for any two); and fruit must not be cooked with sugar (1 mark).

Drinks with no calorie value can be taken freely; these include black coffee, tea with lemon, meat extracts and marmite (2 for any two). Alcohol has a high calorie value, and alcoholic drinks should be avoided if possible (2 marks) or strictly limited (1 mark).

Drugs may be ordered for obesity, but should only be used under medical supervision (1 mark). These include amphetamines (*or* Benzedrine) to reduce the appetite (2 marks), and thyroid extract to speed up the rate of metabolism (2 marks).

Exercise such as walking to work instead of driving may be recommended; but too much exercise may increase the appetite too much (1 mark).

Finally, the patient needs encouragement from her doctor, relations and friends to persevere with her diet; and she may be helped by joining a 'weight-watchers' club' (1 mark).

DISTURBANCES OF METABOLISM
14. Hypothermia

Points to revise

1. Revise the ways in which the body temperature is kept constant.

2. List any groups of individuals who are liable to hypothermia.

3. Make notes on how a patient with hypothermia would be treated in hospital, and on the reasons for this treatment.

4. Make sure you know the reasons for producing hypothermia artificially.

When you have revised these points, and not before, turn over the page.

Question

Without consulting any book, write the answer to the question on this page. You should not take more than 35 minutes to plan and write your answer.

(a)	What do you understand by the term hypothermia?	10%
(b)	What are the causes of this state?	20%
(c)	Describe the nursing care and treatment of a hypothermic patient.	20%
(d)	What use is made of hypothermia in present day treatment?	20%
(e)	How is normal body temperature controlled?	30%

When you have finished your answer, turn over and correct it by the 'model answer' overleaf.

Model answer

(a)   *Hypothermia* (10 marks)

Hypothermia is a condition in which the body temperature is abnormally low (2 marks). The rectal temperature is usually $32°C$ (*or* $90°F$) or lower (5 marks). The patient is often comatose (2 marks), or else drowsy and confused (1 mark).

(b)   *Causes of hypothermia* (20 marks)

It mainly occurs in old people, because the temperature-regulating mechanism is not so efficient in old age (3 marks). Old people can develop hypothermia in cold weather when their houses are not well heated (2 marks). As adequate heating is expensive, their poverty may be a contributing factor (1 mark). It is especially likely if housing is bad or if they have to use an outdoor lavatory or go outside to fetch coal (1 mark); and sometimes results because an old person has an accident or stroke in a cold place, and cannot move for some time (2 marks). A person who is already ill, e.g. with pneumonia, is more likely to suffer from hypothermia (1 mark).

Myxoedemic patients are especially liable to it (2 marks), because lack of thyroxine prevents the normal production of heat and energy (1 mark). It can also occur in new-born babies (2 marks), and especially in premature ones (2 marks), if they are in badly heated rooms (1 mark). In these babies, the heat-regulating mechanism is not yet well developed (1 mark), and they have a relatively large body surface from which heat can be lost (1 mark).

(c)   *Nursing care and treatment* (20 marks)

The patient must not be warmed up suddenly by means of electric blankets or cradles (2 marks). She should be wrapped in blankets so that further heat is not lost (2 marks), and nursed in a warm room with the temperature kept between $26°$ and $32°C$ ($80°$ and $90°F$) (3 marks), so that she warms up gradually (1 mark).

The rectal temperature is taken and charted every hour (2 marks) with a special low-reading thermometer (1 mark).

The patient is usually comatose, so will need turning regularly and all nursing care to prevent development of bedsores (2 marks) and hypostatic pneumonia (1 mark). An antibiotic is usually given to prevent pneumonia (1 mark). Oxygen is also given (1 mark).

The blood pressure is low, so the patient will be given intravenous fluids (2 marks), and hydrocortisone may be added to these (2 marks).

(d) *The use of hypothermia in treatment* (20 marks)

The body temperature may be lowered artificially while heart operations are performed (2 marks). For short operations during which the circulation is stopped for only a few minutes (2 marks), this is done by putting the patient into a bath of iced water (2 marks) while she is under the anaesthetic (1 mark). The body temperature is reduced to 30°C (*or* 86°F) (2 marks). At this temperature the vital organs (*or* brain and kidneys) need less oxygen to keep them alive (5 marks).

For longer operations, when the heart has to be stopped, the temperature is lowered by the heart-lung machine (2 marks), which cools the blood supplied to the body during the operation (2 marks). The temperature is lowered even more, so that vital organs can survive the deficiency of oxygen for longer (2 marks).

(e) *Control of body temperature* (30 marks)

The body temperature is kept constant by a heat-regulating centre in the brain (4 marks). This centre receives nerve impulses from the skin (2 marks), where there are nerve endings sensitive to heat and cold (1 mark). It is also sensitive to the temperature of the blood passing through it (1 mark). In response to these impulses, the centre sends out other nerve impulses to regulate the temperature (1 mark).

As a result, if the body is becoming too hot, the blood vessels in the skin dilate (3 marks), so that heat is lost by radiation (2 marks). The sweat glands produce more sweat (3 marks), and the body is cooled by sweat evaporating from the skin (2 marks). If the body is becoming too cold, loss of heat is prevented (1 mark), because the blood vessels in the skin become constricted (2 marks) and the sweat glands secrete less (2 marks).

The hairs in the skin help to prevent loss of heat by becoming erected when it is cold (2 marks), and so trapping warm air next to the skin (1 mark). Suitable clothing also helps to regulate temperature by keeping in heat or allowing it to escape according to the weather (1 mark). Shivering is an involuntary contraction of muscles (1 mark) which produces heat when the body is cold (1 mark).

DISTURBANCES OF METABOLISM
15. Oedema

Points to revise

1. Make sure you could describe (a) the changes in the tissues which occur in oedema, and (b) how you would recognize oedema.

2. Name conditions which may cause oedema:
   (a) Of one arm
   (b) Of one leg
   (c) Of localized areas in the skin and mucous membranes

3. Make sure you know the reasons why oedema occurs in each of the above conditions.

4. Make sure you can account for the oedema occurring in:
   (a) Congestive heart failure
   (b) Renal disease
   (c) Cirrhosis of the liver
   (d) Severe malnutrition

5. Name any condition of drug treatment which may cause retention of salt in the tissues.

6. Make notes on the kinds of patient for whom fluid balance charts might be kept, and the reasons for keeping them.

When you have revised these points, and not before, turn over the page.

Question

Without consulting any book, write the answer to the question on this page. You should not take more than 35 minutes to plan and write your answer.

(a)	What is oedema?	10%

(b) What are the causes of
  (i) Local oedema   20%
  (ii) Generalized oedema?   20%

(c) Discuss the reasons for keeping fluid balance charts. How would you ensure that these charts are kept accurately?   50%

When you have finished your answer, turn over and correct it by the 'model answer' overleaf.

Model answer

(a)   *Oedema* (10 marks)

Oedema is an accumulation of excess fluid (*or* water) (3 marks) in the tissue spaces (5 marks). It is recognized by 'pitting'; if the skin is pressed, the depression takes some time to disappear (2 marks).

(b)   *Causes of oedema*

(i)   Causes of local oedema (20 marks)

One cause is obstruction of lymphatic vessels (3 marks), e.g. by metastases in lymph nodes (2 marks) or due to surgical removal of lymph nodes (2 marks).

It can also be caused by obstruction of veins (2 marks), by deep venous thrombosis (2 marks) or by pressure from the outside (1 mark), e.g. from a tumour in the pelvis or pregnancy pressing on veins carrying blood from the lower limbs (2 marks for any one example).

Urticaria (1 mark) and angioneurotic oedema (1 mark) are allergic conditions (1 mark) affecting the skin and subcutaneous tissues (1 mark). In conditions causing generalized oedema, the oedema tends at first to be localized in dependent parts of the body (*or* in ankles, sacrum, scrotum) because of gravity (2 marks).

(ii)   Causes of generalized oedema (20 marks)

This is associated specially with renal disease (2 marks), congestive cardiac failure (2 marks) and cirrhosis of the liver (1 mark).

In renal disease it may be due to salt retention, as the kidneys are failing to excrete salt normally (1 mark). In acute nephritis there is also increased permeability of the capillaries (1 mark). Where there is massive albuminuria (*or* proteinuria), there is a lowering of the plasma proteins (2 marks). This lowers the osmotic pressure of the plasma so that fluid escapes from the capillaries (3 marks). This also occurs where there is gross malnutrition, because of lack of protein (2 marks).

In congestive heart failure there is raised blood pressure in the veins due to poor return of blood to the heart, which causes fluid to leak out of the capillaries (3 marks). Cirrhosis of the liver causes raised pressure in the portal system (1 mark).

Salt retention can cause oedema as a result of prolonged treatment with corticosteroids or Cushing's syndrome (2 marks for either).

(c) *Fluid balance charts* (50 marks)

These charts enable doctors and nurses to see if a patient's intake is adequate, and alert them if it is not (2 marks), so that dehydration can be prevented (2 marks). For this reason they are kept for all unconscious patients (1 mark), following operations when the patient may have nothing by mouth (1 mark), and for all ill patients who are not drinking well (1 mark). If the output of urine is insufficient, i.e. less than about 1 litre in 24 hours (1 mark), more fluids must be given, intravenously if necessary (1 mark).

Fluid balance charts must be kept for all patients confined to bed for a long time (*or* any example of this, such as patient with a fractured femur), because of the danger of urinary infection (2 marks) and occasionally the formation of renal calculi (1 mark). They are also kept for patients who have urinary infections (2 marks). A good fluid intake flushes out the kidneys and urinary tract, preventing infection and calculus formation (2 marks). It is especially important if treatment with sulphonamide drugs is used, as these may form crystals which block the renal tubules (1 mark).

A fluid balance chart is kept for any patient with kidney disease (2 marks). The output side will show if oliguria or anuria occurs due to renal failure (1 mark); and an increased output will show that the patient's condition is improving (2 marks). The chart is also required if it is necessary to cut down the fluid intake according to the output of urine (1 mark).

These charts are kept for all patients being treated with diuretics, to see that diuresis is satisfactory (2 marks).

It is especially important to record intake and output after operations on the renal tract (1 mark) or prostate gland (1 mark). One reason is that the patient may develop anuria from renal failure (2 marks); another, that he may get retention of urine due to clots (1 mark). He must also drink plenty in order to prevent urinary infection (1 mark). The same applies to women who have had operations involving the uterus and pelvic floor (1 mark).

A chart should be kept for any severely shocked patient, as acute renal failure may occur due to a low blood pressure (2 marks). The most important instance is with burns (2 marks), when the urine output must be measured every hour at first (1 mark). The amount of intravenous fluid given has to be increased if the output is less than 30 ml each hour (1 mark). As very large amounts of fluid have to be given, it is also essential to make sure that the correct amount runs in (1 mark).

93

To ensure that charts are completed correctly, it is essential that all the nursing staff know exactly which patients are to have intake and output measured (1 mark); and it should be the specific duty of one night nurse and one day nurse to report the totals to the person in charge (1 mark). There must be definite times for adding up the totals (1 mark); usually this will be done in the morning by the night staff and in the evening by the day staff, e.g. at 8 a.m. and 8 p.m. each day (2 marks). All staff should understand that intravenous fluids should be recorded only as each bottle is finished (2 marks) and all other fluid intake immediately after it is taken (2 marks). Urine, vomit or gastric aspiration should be measured and recorded at once, as if a nurse attempts to remember measurements without recording them, they may be inaccurate or forgotten (2 marks).

ALIMENTARY TRACT (2)
16. Difficulty in swallowing

Points to revise

1.   Make notes on:
     (a)   The parts of the nervous system which control swallowing
     (b)   All the structures concerned in swallowing until food
           reaches the stomach

2.   Using the above notes, list the possible causes of dysphagia
     arising through disorders of any of the structures you have
     mentioned.

3.   List any special articles which a nurse might have to provide for
     a doctor examining a patient complaining of dysphagia.

4.   List any observation you would make on this patient after
     admission to the ward.

5.   List any investigations which might be done on the patient,
     together with the nurse's duties in preparing her and caring for
     her following the investigations.

6.   Make notes on
     (a)   The principles involved in planning a diet for a poorly-
           nourished patient suffering from dysphagia
     (b)   Any special methods of feeding which might be
           necessary

When you have revised these points, and not before, turn over the page.

Question

Without consulting any book, write the answer to the question on this page. You should not take more than 35 minutes to plan and write your answer.

Describe the mechanism of swallowing.   20%

An elderly patient is admitted to hospital with difficulty in
swallowing.   20%
(a)   List the causes.   20%
(b)   What observations and investigations may be
       performed on this patient? How may the nurse
       assist in these procedures?   30%
(c)   How would the nurse ensure that this patient
       receives adequate nutrition?   30%

Hint to students: In answering (a), remember the patient's age, and confine yourself to causes likely at that time of life.

When you have finished your answer, turn over and correct it by the 'model answer' overleaf.

Model answer

The mechanism of swallowing (20 marks)

The mechanism of swallowing is controlled by the glossopharyngeal (*or* ninth cranial) nerve (2 marks), which arises in the medulla oblongata of the brain (2 marks).

Solid food which has been masticated (1 mark) and moistened by saliva (1 mark) is rolled into a bolus by the tongue (1 mark), and pushed back by the tongue into the pharynx (1 mark). The muscles of the pharynx close on it (2 marks) and pass it down to the oesophagus (1 mark). In the oesophagus it is passed down by peristalsis (2 marks). The cardiac sphincter relaxes to allow it to pass into the stomach (2 marks).

During swallowing the soft palate rises and shuts off the nasopharynx (2 marks). The larynx rises (1 mark), so that the epiglottis closes over it to prevent food from entering the air passages (2 marks).

(a) Causes of difficulty in swallowing (20 marks)

In an elderly patient, these might be:

Bulbar paralysis (2 marks), probably due to a cerebrovascular accident (*or* stroke) (3 marks)

Quinsy (2 marks)

Carcinoma of oesophagus (4 marks) or larynx (2 marks)

Pressure from mediastinal tumour (*or* carcinoma of bronchus) (2 marks for either)

Cardiospasm (*or* achalasia of the cardia) (3 marks)

Hiatus hernia (2 marks).

(b) Observations and investigations (30 marks)

The doctor will first examine the patient, and the nurse will stay with him to help and to reassure the patient while this is happening (1 mark). Depending on the suspected causes, the nurse may have to provide for the doctor a torch and spatula for examining the throat (1 mark), and for examination of the larynx a laryngoscope (1 mark) and spray containing local anaesthetic (1 mark) (*or* 2 marks for laryngeal mirror and spirit lamp). In case the suspected cause is a cerebrovascular accident (1 mark), she will provide an ophthalmoscope (1 mark), patella hammer (1 mark) and sphygnomanometer and stethoscope (1 mark).

When the patient is in the ward, the nurse must keep a fluid balance chart (2 marks). This will show how much fluid the patient is taking (1 mark), and will also record any occasions on which she regurgitates

or vomits food (1 mark). A close watch must also be kept on any solid food which she takes and whether this is regurgitated (1 mark). The nurse should also notice and report any complaints of discomfort or pain from the patient (1 mark). A record of the patient's weight will be kept to see if she is gaining weight under treatment (1 mark).
A barium swallow may be done (2 marks) in order to detect carcinoma of the oesophagus (1 mark), and also to see whether the cardiac sphincter is functioning normally (*or* to detect cardiospasm) (1 mark). The nurse must see that the patient has nothing to eat overnight before the examination (1 mark), and that she has an aperient afterwards to clear out the barium (1 mark).
Oesophagoscopy may be done (2 marks). Again, the patient should have nothing by mouth overnight (1 mark). The nurse may have to give the patient local anaesthetic tablets before she goes to theatre (1 mark), and should explain to her that she must suck, and not swallow, them (2 marks). Following oesophagoscopy, the patient should have nothing by mouth for 2–4 hours until her swallowing reflex returns (2 marks). She should then be given sips of water before being given anything else by mouth, and any pain should be reported, in case there is any damage to the oesophagus (1 mark).

(d) *Ensuring that the patient receives adequate nutrition* (30 marks)

This patient will probably have lost weight, so will require a high-calorie diet (2 marks). The dietician (*or* catering officer) should be consulted, so that a suitable diet can be planned (2 marks). The patient herself should also be consulted as to what foods she likes and finds easiest to swallow (2 marks). Usually patients with dysphagia find it easier to swallow thickened fluids rather than thinner ones (1 mark) and semi-solids rather than solids (1 mark). Suitable foods might be milk thickened with Complan or arrowroot, egg custards, milk jellies, thick soups and mince (3 marks for any 3 examples).
The patient must be encouraged to eat her diet (2 marks), and not hurried (2 marks). The nurse must point it out to the doctor if she is not eating well (1 mark), if her fluid intake is too little (1 mark) or if she is losing weight (1 mark). The nurse may also have to show the patient how to pass weighted oesophageal bougies which dilate the cardiac sphincter before each meal (1 mark).
A milk drip may be set up to supplement the diet (2 marks). In this case the nurse should make sure that the required amount runs in

through the nasogastric tube (1 mark) — probably two or three pints in 24 hours (1 mark).

The patient may have to be fed artificially through a nasogastric tube (1 mark), or, if the oesophageal carcinoma is advanced, through a gastro-stomy opening (1 mark). The feeds may consist of Complan (1 mark) or of a special mixture based on milk (1 mark). These will contain all the necessary food factors in fluid form (1 mark) and will provide 2000—3000 calories a day (1 mark). The nurse must make sure that the correct amounts are given at the correct times (1 mark).

ALIMENTARY TRACT
17. Haematemesis

Points to revise

1. Make sure you know the meaning of the term 'haematemesis' and could give reasons why it occurs.

2. List the observations you would make on a patient who has had a haematemesis, and the investigations which may be ordered by the doctor.

3. Make notes on what can be learnt from the observations you have mentioned.

4. How might this patient be treated:
    (a) Medically (or conservatively)
    (b) Surgically

When you have revised these points, and not before, turn over the page.

Question

Without consulting any book, write the answer to the question on this page. You should not take more than 35 minutes to plan and write your answer.

A patient has been admitted to hospital after having a large haematemesis.

(a) What observations would you make on admission and why are these important? 40%

(b) What immediate investigations will be performed? 10%

(c) Discuss the nursing care and treatment of the emergency. 40%

(d) List the causes of haematemesis. 10%

When you have finished your answer, turn over and correct it by the 'model answer' overleaf.

Model answer

(a) *Observations and their importance* (40 marks)

The patient's general condition must be assessed so that comparison can be made later; it should be noticed whether he is alert or seems confused (3 marks). If he suddenly becomes confused, it probably means that the bleeding is continuing and he is suffering from cerebral anoxia (2 marks). Worry and anxiety adds to his state of unease, and he can be reassured, which may help to calm him (2 marks).

His temperature, pulse, respiration rate and blood pressure should be taken and recorded. Charts are made out for the patient (5 marks). The pulse will be taken and charted every 15–30 minutes; any rise will indicate further haemorrhage. Blood pressure will be taken every half an hour, and if the systolic pressure falls below 90 mm Hg, the foot of the bed should be elevated and the doctor notified as this, too, means bleeding is taking place (5 marks).

Respirations will probably be shallow, and if these change to sighing (*or* 'air hunger') this is another sign of bleeding (2 marks).

If the patient suddenly becomes restless it is another indication of bleeding and doctor should be informed (4 marks).

The patient's colour will also be a guide to change in his condition: if he becomes paler or ashen-grey it is a sign of deterioration; if he becomes cyanosed he will need to be given oxygen because of lack of blood (4 marks).

If the patient complains of nausea or vomits, a nasogastric tube is passed so that his stomach can be kept empty and the aspirate can be frequently observed for fresh blood. It will also save the patient the distress and exertion of vomiting (6 marks).

Should the patient have a bowel action, the amount and appearance of the stool should be noted: if the bleeding continues, the stools may be frequent and large and will be black and tarry (*or* melaena) because they contain altered blood (3 marks).

The patient may start to complain of pain or discomfort, and the nurse should notice whether this improves with rest. It may only be a symptom if the stomach is allowed to fill with blood without being aspirated; aspiration of the stomach by tube may relieve the pain; this should be reported also (4 marks).

(b) *Immediate investigations* (10 marks)

Blood will be taken for haemoglobin estimation (2 marks) and for grouping and cross-matching as a blood transfusion will be needed (4 marks).

The patient's urine will be tested for abnormalities and the results recorded, as emergency surgery may have to be performed (3 marks). If the patient is fit enough, he may have a small barium meal so the stomach can be X-rayed (1 mark).

(c) *Nursing care and treatment* (40 marks)

This patient is best nursed flat in bed with one soft pillow under his head (2 marks); the pillow should be protected by a waterproof cover or protective (1 mark).

The doctor will order a hypnotic such as morphine or papaveretum (Omnopon) to help the patient to rest; this should be given by intra-muscular injection as soon as possible (5 marks).

He should be disturbed as little as possible, and nurses must not appear to be anxious or in a hurry when attending to the patient (2 marks). Sponging his hands and face will add to his comfort (1 mark).

The patient will be allowed nothing to eat or drink at first (2 marks). His dentures should be taken out, cleaned and put in a labelled container; he will appreciate a mouthwash such as lemon and soda, or glycerin of thymol, and he should be helped with this (3 marks). He may be allowed ice to suck (1 mark).

Quarter or half-hourly observations are continued; the foot of the bed is raised if he shows signs of shock and lowered if his condition improves (*or* if his pulse decreases and his blood pressure rises) (3 marks). Any changes are reported, as, if bleeding continues or starts again, emergency operation (*or* emergency partial gastrectomy) will be performed (4 marks).

An intravenous infusion will be set up. Normal saline or dextrose in saline will probably be given at first; later blood will be given but this is allowed to flow in slowly to avoid raising the patient's blood pressure too rapidly and restarting the bleeding (6 marks).

A fluid balance chart is recorded (1 mark).

Some doctors like the patient to be given a diluted milk 'drip' via the nasogastric tube, or small hourly feeds of diluted milk, as soon as the patient no longer feels nauseated; other doctors like a soft diet to be started very early in treatment (allow 4 marks for giving a method of feeding that you have seen employed).

The patient's relatives should be seen by the doctor, or nurse in charge of the ward, and should be told about the patient's condition (2 marks).

The possibility of an operation is also explained and they should be asked to sign the operation consent form, to prevent worrying the patient (2 marks). If there are social problems, the medical social worker is asked to see the patient or his relatives (1 mark).

(d)   *Causes of haematemesis* (10 marks)

Peptic (*or* gastric) ulcer which erodes a blood vessel in the stomach wall (2 marks).

Oesophageal varices caused by portal hypertension (*or* hepatic cirrhosis) (2 marks).

Carcinoma of stomach (1 mark).

Administration of anticoagulants (2 marks), aspirin (2 marks) or corticosteroids (1 mark).

ALIMENTARY TRACT (2)
18. Perforated Peptic Ulcer

Points to revise

1. Make sure you could describe the signs and symptoms of a patient who had a perforated peptic ulcer, and that you know the dangers of this condition.

2. List any signs which would make you suspect that his condition was deteriorating.

3. List the essential points in:
   (a) The preoperative treatment
   (b) The postoperative treatment and nursing care of a patient with perforated peptic ulcer.

When you have revised these points, and not before, turn over the page.

Question

Without consulting any book, write the answer to the question on this page. You should not take more than 35 minutes to plan and write your answer.

A young man is admitted to hospital with perforated peptic ulcer.

(a)	What observations would you make on this patient on admission?	20%
(b)	Describe the preparation of this patient for operation.	40%
(c)	Describe the specific postoperative nursing care of this patient.	40%

When you have finished your answer, turn over and correct it by the 'model answer' overleaf.

Model answer

(a) *Observations of admission* (20 marks)

Signs of shock should be noticed (1 mark): whether the skin is cold and perspiring (1 mark) and whether the patient is pale and anxious-looking (1 mark). His temperature, pulse and respiration will be taken (1 mark); and a quarter- or half-hourly pulse chart started (1 mark). I would notice whether the pulse was feeble (1 mark), and whether it was becoming more rapid (1 mark). The patient's blood-pressure would also be taken and charted (1 mark). I should also notice whether his abdominal muscles, or only his chest muscles, moved during respiration (1 mark). I should notice whether the patient appeared to be in great pain, or complained of pain (2 marks), or whether he was pain-free but becoming lethargic (1 mark).

It would also be important to notice if his abdomen started to become distended (2 marks), or if he began to vomit (2 marks), as these are signs of advanced peritonitis (1 mark). It should also be noticed whether vomiting is effortless (1 mark), and whether the vomit is bile-stained (1 mark). A pinched look about his face and sunken eyes would also be noticed if the peritonitis was advanced (1 mark).

(b) *Preparation for operation* (40 marks)

The patient will need to be prepared for theatre as quickly as possible (2 marks). He should be asked when he last had anything to eat or drink (3 marks), and a nasogastric tube will be passed, and any stomach contents aspirated (3 marks). The tube will be left in position when he goes to the theatre (1 mark).

He must be told that an operation is essential (1 mark), and reassured as much as possible that he will recover quickly once he had had it (2 marks). The form for consent to operation must be explained to him (1 mark), and he must sign it (2 marks).

Because of his shocked condition, he must be taken to the ward and lifted into bed with great gentleness (2 marks); and then should be moved as little as possible until he goes to the theatre, so only the essential preparation is undertaken (1 mark).

He must be given a urinal and asked to provide a specimen of urine (1 mark). This is tested for abnormalities (1 mark), and the result written in his notes (2 marks).

He will probably have had an injection of an analgesic such as morphine as soon as his condition was diagnosed (2 marks); and further premedication of atropine or scopolamine will be ordered (2 marks). This is checked and given if possible about 45 minutes before he goes to the theatre (2 marks).

The abdomen should be washed only if it is very dirty (1 mark); and if possible the abdomen and pubic area should be shaved (2 marks), though this may be done in the theatre if he is very snocked (1 mark). He is dressed in theatre gown and socks (2 marks), and an identity bracelet is attached to his wrist or ankle (2 marks). Any dentures or prostheses are removed (2 marks). He should then be kept very quiet until the theatre trolley arrives (1 mark), and a nurse should accompany him to the theatre to reassure him (1 mark).

(c) *Specific postoperative nursing care* (40 marks)

On his return from the theatre the patient will have a nasogastric tube in position (1 mark), and may have a drainage tube in his abdominal wound (1 mark). An intravenous infusion will be in progress (1 mark). The nasogastric tube must be aspirated frequently (2 marks), and the amounts aspirated entered on a fluid balance chart (2 marks). The nurses must see that the correct amounts and kinds of intravenous fluid are given according to the doctor's instructions (2 marks), and that the infusion is running correctly (1 mark). These fluids will also be entered on his fluid chart (1 mark). He will have nothing by mouth until the doctor has heard bowel sounds (2 marks), and until the amount of fluid aspirated has diminished (1 mark). As he is taking nothing by mouth, he will need to have his mouth cleaned or to use mouthwashes (1 mark).

A postoperative analgesic will be ordered, and is given as soon as necessary to prevent pain (1 mark); it may be repeated according to the doctor's instructions (1 mark).

He should be propped up in bed to prevent any fluid in the abdomen from collecting under the diaphragm (2 marks). His wound must be observed frequently at first, and the amount and character of drainage from the tube reported (2 marks). The dressing should be re-packed or changed if it becomes soaked with fluid or blood (1 mark). The drainage tube will be removed when no further fluid is leaking out (1 mark); and the stitches are removed after about 10 days (1 mark). The patient will be taught breathing exercises, which the nursing staff must encourage him to practise (2 marks). He should be sat out of bed for a short time on the day after operation, and will then be allowed up for longer periods each day (1 mark).

Once bowel sounds have been heard, the nasogastric tube is removed
(1 mark), and the patient is given gradually increasing quantities of
water, probably starting with 30 ml each hour. (2 marks). After 12—24
hours, he will be given milk and other fluids freely (2 marks); the
intravenous infusion will then be discontinued provided he does not
vomit (1 mark). The next day he will be given a light gastric diet
(2 marks), and by the end of a week will be having a full gastric diet
(1 mark).

He will probably be discharged after 2 weeks (1 mark); and will be
advised not to smoke (1 mark), to have no alcohol or other foods
which give him indigestion and to eat small regular meals (1 mark). He
should understand that his own doctor will tell him when he may return
to work (1 mark).

Points to revise

1. Make sure you could give an account of the structure of the kidney.

2. List the organs which lie near the kidneys.

3. List the investigations which may be undertaken for a patient with a tumour of one kidney.

4. Make sure you could describe the specific postoperative care required for patients after operations on the kidney.

When you have revised these points, and not before, turn over the page.

Question

Without comsulting any book, write the answer to the question on this page. You should not take more than 35 minutes to plan and write your answer.

A patient is admitted with suspected carcinoma of one kidney.

(a)	Describe the anatomy and immediate relations of the right kidney.	30%
(b)	What investigations may be required in this condition?	20%
(c)	Describe the specific nursing care following nephrectomy.	50%

When you have finished your answer, turn over and correct it by the 'model answer' overleaf.

Model answer

(a) *Anatomy and relations of the right kidney* (30 marks)

The kidney is a bean-shaped organ (1 mark) lying on the right side of the posterior part of the abdominal cavity (1 mark), behind the peritoneum (1 mark). It is parallel to the upper 3 lumbar vertebrae (1 mark). The kidney is supplied with blood by the renal artery (1 mark) which branches off the abdominal aorta (1 mark); the artery enters the kidney at the hilum (1 mark). The renal vein (1 mark) leaves by way of the hilum and empties its contents into the inferior vena cava (1 mark). The right ureter also leaves the kidney at the hilum, carrying urine to the bladder (1 mark).

The kidney lies embedded in fat (1 mark) and is surrounded by a fibrous capsule (1 mark).

The outer part of the kidney, the cortex (1 mark) consists of about 1 million nephrons (1 mark) with their surrounding blood capillaries (1 mark). The middle part, the medulla (1 mark), consists of collecting tubules (*or* collecting ducts) (1 mark), forming the pyramids (1 mark). These drain into the central hollow called the kidney pelvis (1 mark), which is lined with epithelium (1 mark) continuous with that lining the ureter and bladder (1 mark). Branches of the pelvis are the calyces (1 mark) which act as funnels through which urine drains (1 mark).

Other relations. Above the kidney is the adrenal (or supra-renal) gland (1 mark); across the top of the kidney is the liver (1 mark); behind is the posterior abdominal wall (*or* lumbar muscles) (1 mark); in front lie the ascending (1 mark), hepatic flexure (1 mark) and transverse colon (1 mark) and loops of small intestine (1 mark).

(b) *Investigations* (20 marks)

The patient's urine will be tested on the ward for abnormalities, particularly blood and albumin (3 marks).

A mid-stream specimen of urine will be sent to the laboratory to be examined for blood cells and bacteriological culture (2 marks).

The patient's haemoglobin and blood urea will be estimated (2 marks), and blood will be grouped and cross-matched for the operation (2 marks).

A straight X-ray of the abdomen will be taken (2 marks), and an intravenous pyelogram will be performed (3 marks). Retrograde pyelography may also be necessary (2 marks). An aortogram, or renal arteriogram, may also be done (2 marks).

A chest X-ray will be taken to exclude metastases (2 marks).

(c) *Specific postoperative care after nephrectomy* (50 marks)

In the immediate postoperative period the patient must be observed for signs of shock and reactionary haemorrhage (2 marks) and his pulse and blood pressure should be taken and recorded half-hourly (2 marks). His intravenous infusion, or blood transfusion, should be observed and maintained according to the surgeon's instructions (2 marks).

To facilitate drainage, the patient should be placed in bed leaning over to the side of operation (3 marks), with protected pillows placed down his back for support (2 marks).

Drainage will probably be of the 'Redivac' type, in which case the amount is measured and charted each day when the bottle is changed. If the drainage becomes very heavily blood-stained, it should be reported to the doctor (3 marks). *Alternatively*, if there is a corrugated drain tube, the dressing may need repacking during the first 24 hours, after which the area around the tube will require redressing once or twice daily. If drainage seems excessive, or is very heavily blood-stained, it should be reported (3 marks for *this* method).

The drain is removed when drainage has lessened, usually about the 4th or 5th postoperative day (2 marks).

As soon as possible, fluids are given by mouth and the patient is encouraged to drink 2–2½ litres per day (2 marks). A fluid balance chart is recorded (2 marks). It should be reported if the patient does not pass urine by 12–15 hours after operation (2 marks) or if the urinary output is not adequate (2 marks). The intravenous infusion will be discontinued when the fluid intake is satisfactory (1 mark).

During the first week, the patient should be observed for signs of uraemia, and it should be reported if he seems drowsy or dehydrated (3 marks). A dry, brown-coated tongue is another sign which can be observed by the nursing staff and reported (2 marks).

A 4-hourly temperature, pulse and respiration chart is kept and any rises are regarded as being indicative of chest or wound infection (3 marks). Deep venous thrombosis may cause a slight rise of temperature about 5–7 days after operation (2 marks).

Adequate analgesics should be given for the first 48 hours as the patient will find it painful to move about and to practice his breathing exercises and leg movements (3 marks). He will be helped out of bed for bedmaking, if he is well enough, the day after operation (1 mark). After this, mobilization can be increased daily (1 mark).

Stitches can usually be removed 8—12 days postoperatively (2 marks). The patient may be apprehensive about his future if he suspects he has malignant disease, and some form of diversional therapy should be available (2 marks). He should be encouraged to mix with the other patients in the day-room (2 marks).

Relatives should be seen by the doctor and the patient's condition discussed with them; they should also be told if treatment is to be continued by radiotherapy (2 marks).

Convalescence may be advised before further treatment is undertaken or it may be delayed until treatment is finished (2 marks).

URINARY SYSTEM (2)
20. Renal Colic

Points to revise

1. Make sure you could describe an attack of severe colic.

2. List the different organs in which colic originates.

3. Name any drugs which are used to treat severe colic.

4. Make some notes on the treatment of a patient with renal colic.

5. In a case of renal colic, list the ways in which treatment may differ according to the position of the calculus.

When you have revised these points, and not before, turn over the page.

Question

Without consulting any book, write the answer to the question on this page. You should not take more than 35 minutes to plan and write your answer.

Explain what is meant by 'colic'. List the different types of colic.   20%

A young man is admitted with renal colic.
   (a)   What may be the cause of this?   10%

   (b)   What signs and symptoms will be present?   10%

   (c)   Describe his immediate treatment and nursing care.   30%

   (d)   Outline the further treatment which may be required.   30%

When you have finished your answer, turn over and correct it by the 'model answer' overleaf.

Model answer

Colic (20 marks)

Colic means severe pain (2 marks) which is spasmodic (2 marks). It occurs when the muscular walls of hollow tubes contract violently (3 marks), usually in an attempt to expel something in the lumen (3 marks).

Types of colic
Renal colic (1 mark)
Gallstone (*or* biliary) colic (3 marks)
Salivary colic (1 mark)
Intestinal colic (3 marks)
Appendicular colic (1 mark)
Tubal (*or* Fallopian tube) colic (1 mark)

(a) *Cause of renal colic* (10 marks)

The usual cause is renal calculus (*or* a stone in the urinary tract) (5 marks). The muscular wall of the ureter (2 marks) tries to push the stone downwards, by peristalsis, to the bladder (3 marks).

(b) *Signs and symptoms* (10 marks)

The patient will complain of severe pain in the loin (2 marks) which radiates round to the groin (1 mark) and may also be felt at the tip of the penis (1 mark). The pain comes and goes (1 mark).
The pulse will be rapid (1 mark) and there may be pallor and sweating during the attack (2 marks).
The pain may be so severe that the patient rolls about (1 mark) and he may vomit (1 mark).

(c) *Immediate treatment and nursing care* (30 marks)

The patient should be put to bed in any position that is comfortable (1 mark).
The application of heat such as by means of a hot water bottle or electric pad may be comforting (2 marks).
The doctor will order an antispasmodic drug, probably to be given by injection (2 marks) and repeated 4- or 6-hourly (1 mark). Examples are: pethidine, methadone (Physeptone), morphine and atropine or propantheline (Pro-Banthine) (4 marks for any 2 examples). Later analgesics may be sufficient, when the colicky pain has ceased, for example: paracetamol, codeine, dihydrocodeine tartrate (*or* D.F.118) (1 for any 1 example).

The patient should be urged to drink copiously, at least 2½—3 litres in 24 hours (4 marks). These can be given in any form that he likes (1 mark). A fluid balance chart should be kept to make sure he is drinking enough and passing adequate amounts of urine (2 marks). His urine should be tested for abnormalities, particularly for blood and albumin; the results should be recorded on his chart (3 marks). A straight X-ray of renal tract will be performed, and if the stone is visible this may be repeated to see if it has moved (3 marks). An intravenous pyelogram may also be performed (2 marks).

All urine passed must be strained for the stones (5 marks).

(d) *Further treatment* (30 marks)

The patient should stay in bed until his spasmodic pain has stopped; he can then get up and be about the ward as he wishes (2 marks). He should continue to drink large amounts of fluids (2 marks). The patient's urine should still be strained (2 marks), and tested daily for blood and albumin (2 marks). A mid-stream specimen will be obtained and sent to the laboratory for bacteriological culture and antibiotic sensitivity (2 marks); if necessary the patient will be given a 7—10 day course of the appropriate antibiotic (*or* ampicillin, sulphamethizole (Urolucosil) or nitrofurantoin) (2 marks). If further X-rays show the calculus still to be present, treatment will depend on its position (1 mark).

If situated at the *ureteric junction* with the bladder (1 mark), an operating cystoscope will be passed under a general anaesthetic and the stone removed under direct vision (2 marks). The patient goes home when there is no haematuria or other symptoms (2 marks).

If in the *bladder*, cystoscopy will show its exact position (1 mark), and the stone may be crushed with a lithotrite (2 marks). After this the bladder is washed out (2 marks). The patient will most likely be fit enough for discharge the next day (1 mark).

If the stone remains in the *ureter* (1 mark), a ureterolithotomy is performed (2 marks); a drainage tube is left in the ureter while any oedema subsides (2 marks). The patient's postoperative care is as for any other major renal tract surgery (1 mark).

URINARY SYSTEM (2)
21. Acute Renal Failure

Points to revise

1. Make sure that you know the possible causes of renal failure. It
    may help to classify these under the following headings:
    (a) Pre-renal causes (i.e. causes not caused by any disease of
         the renal tract)
    (b) Renal causes
    (c) Post-renal causes

2. (a) List the equipment required when a doctor is going to set
         up a peritoneal dialysis.
    (b) Make notes on any preparation which the patient requires
         for this.

3. Make sure you know the nurse's duties while peritoneal dialysis
    is in progress:
    (a) In managing the equipment.
    (b) In making observations
    (c) In caring for the patient

The following articles in back numbers of the *Nursing Times* would be
useful reading: An article on a renal unit, and a case study, 'Terminal
renal failure', 3rd April, 1969; and a series, 'Substitution of kidney
function by artificial means', 18th and 25th September and 2nd and 9th
October, 1969. *Plug in for Life* by Keith Bill, published by Oliphant, is a
book about dialysis from the patient's angle.

When you have revised these points, and not before, turn over the page.

Question

Without consulting any book, write the answer to the question on this page. You should not take more than 35 minutes to plan and write your answer.

A patient in a general ward has acute renal failure and is to have peritoneal dialysis.

(a) List the causes of acute renal failure. 20%

(b) Describe the observations you would make, and the nursing care you would give, to a patient having peritoneal dialysis. 50%

(c) What other forms of treatment might be used if this measure fails, and what problems may arise in connection with these treatments? 30%

When you have finished your answer, turn over and correct it by the 'model answer' overleaf.

Model answer

(a)   *Causes of acute renal failure* (20 marks)

Loss of circulating fluid (2 marks) due to:
> Severe haemorrhage (2 marks)
> Burns (2 marks)
> Shock (1 mark) for example from crush injuries or major operations (1 mark for either example)
> Dehydration (2 marks) for example from profuse diarrhoea or vomiting (1 mark for either)

Back pressure on the kidneys (2 marks) due to:
> Bladder neck obstruction (*or* any cause of this such as enlarged prostate gland or congenital urethral valves) (1 mark)
> Obstruction or damage to the ureters (1 mark) caused by bilateral renal calculi, growths in the abdomen or accidental damage to ureters during operation (1 mark for any example)

Acute glomeruler nephritis (2 marks)

Damage to the kidneys by toxins (*or* septicaemia) (1 mark), or blockage of the tubules due to agglutination of red blood cells by an incompatible blood transfusion or drugs such as sulphonamides or gold (1 for any 1 example).

(b)   *Observations and nursing care* (50 marks)

The nurse must explain to the patient what is to be done (1 mark), and reassure her by saying that she will be given a local anaesthetic, so she will not feel anything but the first prick (1 mark).

The abdomen is shaved from umbilicus to pubis (2 marks), and the bladder must be empty before the procedure (2 marks); so it will probably be necessary to catheterize the patient. A sedative may be ordered, which will be given an hour before the procedure (1 mark). The containers of dialysing fluid are warmed to body temperature in warm water (1 mark). When the apparatus has been set up, the nurse must make sure that the fluid runs in at the correct rate (2 marks). When it has run in, she clamps off the tubing leading to the abdomen (1 mark), and sees that the fluid remains in the peritoneal cavity for the exact time ordered (2 marks). She then allows the fluid to drain out (1 mark), either by lowering the containers on to the floor, so that it siphons back (2 marks), or by releasing a clamp which leads to another drainage bag (2 marks).

When the drainage stops, the tubing is clamped off (1 mark), and the amount recorded (2 marks), together with the amount of fluid which ran in (1 mark).

Further containers of dialysing fluid must be warmed before they are put up (1 mark), and some fluid is run into the drip chamber so that air does not enter the peritoneal cavity (1 mark). Aseptic precautions must be taken when removing or putting up containers (2 marks).

The dressing round the cannula must be kept covered, and replaced if there is any leakage (2 marks). The patient is kept as comfortable as possible; as he cannot move, he could be nursed on a ripple bed or air-ring (1 mark); and his position should be changed each time the dialysis is completed (1 mark).

A fluid balance chart will be kept (2 marks), and any improvement in urine output reported (2 marks). Any urine passed is tested for specific gravity (1 mark) and albumin (1 mark). The amount of fluid permitted by mouth may be restricted according to the urine output (2 marks): 500 ml plus the amount of the previous day's output (1 mark). If the patient is able to eat, protein in the diet is restricted to about 40 g per day (1 mark). If she is too ill to take anything by mouth, intravenous infusion of low protein high calorie food may be given (1 mark); and the nurse must see that the correct amount runs in over the correct period of time (1 mark).

A patient with acute renal failure will be very ill, and will need constant attention (1 mark). The mouth becomes very dry, and must be cleaned frequently (2 marks). There is a possiblity of heart failure and pulmonary oedema (1 mark), so the nurse must notice and report breathlessness (1 mark) or 'bubbly' respirations (1 mark). There also might be a sudden drop in blood pressure due to loss of fluid from the dialysis (1 mark); so she should report any changes in pulse or blood pressure (1 mark).

(c)   *Other forms of treatment* (30 marks)

If the condition becomes chronic, the patient may have to have haemo-dialysis (*or* be put on a kidney machine) (3 marks). This will have to be done two or three times every week for the rest of her life (1 mark). Problems connected with this treatment are:

    (a)   Shortage of beds in special units (1 mark).
    (b)   Disruption of the patient's life from having to spend two nights

each week in the unit (2 marks), which leads to much psycho-logical stress (1 mark).
(c)   Risks of sepsis from the shunt (1 mark), and of serum jaundice (1 mark). There is also a risk to the staff of contracting jaundice (1 mark).

If the patient has a machine at home, problems are:
(a)   Alterations necessary to the house in order to accommodate the apparatus (1 mark), which requires a special room (1 mark), with running water (1 mark), electric power points (1 mark) and telephone (1 mark).
(b)   Training the patient and a relative to work the machine (1 mark), sterilize equipment (1 mark) and cope with emergencies (1 mark); all of which requires intelligence and a stable personality (1 mark).

Another possible treatment is a kidney transplant (3 marks). Problems are that of obtaining a kidney of the right tissue type (2 marks); and that even if this is found the patient may 'reject' it (2 marks). She has to take anti-immune drugs, which destory her resistance to infection (3 marks).

22. RADIOTHERAPY

This chapter is mainly suitable for those students who have worked in a Radiotherapy Department, or who have visited a Centre recently.

Points to revise

1. List some of the conditions treated by radiotherapy.

2. Make sure you know what methods are employed to treat patients:
   (a) By deep X-rays
   (b) By gamma rays

3. What are the dangers in a Radiotherapy Department to:
   (a) The patients
   (b) The staff
   List the dangers and the steps taken to prevent them.

4. Make some notes on the special nursing care required by patients undergoing radiotherapy, with regard to:
   (a) Their psychological requirements
   (b) Their general requirements

5. List the reactions which may occur during treatment affecting:
   (a) The skin
   (b) The general health of the patient
   Make some notes on how these reactions can be prevented and treated.

When you have revised these points, and not before, turn over the page.

Question

Without consulting any book, write the answer to the question on this page. You should not take more than 35 minutes to plan and write your answer

(a)	What do you understand by the term 'radiotherapy'?	10%
(b)	Discuss the forms in which radiotherapy may be given.	20%
(c)	What special precautions are necessary with this form of treatment?	20%
(d)	Describe the nursing care of a patient who is receiving radiotherapy for carcinoma of breast.	50%

When you have finished your answer, turn over and correct it by the 'model answer' overleaf.

Model answer

(a) *Radiotherapy* (10 marks)

This means the employment of radiation (2 marks) by means of deep
X-rays (1 mark), or radium (*or* gamma rays) (1 mark) to treat certain
diseases.

A sufficient dose is given to kill abnormal tissue cells (2 marks) without
damaging healthy ones (1 mark).

Radiotherapy is mostly used for treating malignant conditions (2 marks),
but it can also be used in other diseases such as keloid scarring, spon-
dylosis and birth-marks (1 mark for any 1 example).

(b) *Forms in which radiotherapy is given* (20 marks)

Deep X-rays. Used in low voltage to treat superficial lesions such as skin
cancers (2 marks).

By means of modern linear accelerators, high voltage beams can be
directed on to more deep-seated tumours (2 marks) such as those of
the bladder, breast or lung (1 mark for any 1 example).

Radium. This emits gamma rays and can be enclosed in thin, hollow
needles (1 mark) or specially shaped applicators (1 mark). In this form,
radiotherapy is used for cancers of the tongue (1 mark), cervix (1 mark),
skin or palate (1 mark for either).

Another way of using radium is by drawing off its gas, called radon,
into thin glass tubes known as radon seeds (1 mark) which are placed
in the tissues at operation (1 mark).

Radioactive cobalt, used in a machine, gives a powerful beam of gamma
radiation (1 mark).

Radioactive Isotopes. Certain substances such as iodine, phosphorus and
gold can be made radioactive in an atomic pile (1 mark).

These can be used diagnostically by introducing them into the body and
measuring their uptake by certain organs, e.g. the thyroid gland will
take up radioactive iodine (1 mark). They are also used to locate the
position of some tumours using a Geiger counter, e.g. in the brain or
liver (1 mark for either).

In blood diseases, they are used to ascertain the survival time of red
cells (1 mark); radioactive phosphorus is used on the bone marrow in
the treatment of polycythaemia, thrombocytopaenia and leukaemia
(1 mark for any 1 example).

Radioactive gold can be introduced into the peritioneal, or pleural,
cavity to cause adhesions to prevent malignant ascites and pleural
effusion (2 marks).

(c)   *Special precautions* (20 marks)

Unless enclosed in lead-lined containers, any radioactive substance can affect anyone coming in contact with it (1 mark). Various precautions are taken in wards and departments to minimize this hazard: patients with radium implants are kept in bed away from other patients; the bed is labelled to keep other people away (1 mark). Nurses should keep at least 10 feet away from the bed, and when performing essential treatment on the patient must do so quickly (1 mark). Nurses wear film badges which will indicate if they are receiving too much radiation (1 mark); permanent ward staff have frequent blood tests for the same reason (1 mark).

To protect healthy tissues, very careful dosage (1 mark), positioning of the radium, or X-ray beams (1 mark) and length of time of treatment are worked out by the doctor (1 mark). The doctor also marks out the fields on the skin so that the radiotherapists can carry out the treatment (1 mark).

Radium itself is in very short supply and very expensive, and these are additional reasons for safeguarding it (1 mark). A trained person is in charge of its lead-lined safe (1 mark).

A register is kept with particulars about each patient for whom it is used (1 mark), with the dose (1 mark). The book is signed by the theatre sister who receives the radium (1 mark), and by the doctor who removes it at the conclusion of treatment (1 mark). It is carefully checked before being put back into the safe (1 mark).

Radium is handled by staff wearing gloves (1 mark) and by long-handled forceps (1 mark). It is transported to and from the patient in lead-lined containers with long handles to keep it well away from the person carrying it (1 mark).

Any loss of radium, or other radioactive materials, is reported at once (1 mark).

(d)   *Nursing care* (50 marks)

The patient will almost certainly know her diagnosis and she should be given a great deal of hope and reassurance about the successful outcome of her treatment (2 marks). She may have already undergone surgery, or is having treatment prior to operation: in either case, she will need comforting about her appearance (2 marks). A nurse must take time to explain what radiotherapy treatment involves (1 mark), assuring her that all she will have to do is to lie still for a few minutes (1 mark), and that she will feel no pain (2 marks). A nurse she knows should go with her to the department for her first treatment (2 marks).

If the patient is well enough, she should be up and dressed (2 marks) and have some form of diversional or occupational therapy (1 mark). An openbacked gown may be the easiest for her to wear for treatment (1 mark). Visitors should be encouraged to come to see her and, as the radiotherapy centre may be a distance from her home, financial assistance may be able to be arranged to help with fares (2 marks). The patient should be helped by the nurses to take a pride in her personal appearance and should make use of any facilities provided, such as hairdressing (2 marks).

While receiving treatment, the patient should have a good diet with plenty of protein (2 marks); her fluid intake should be 2—2½ litres per day to help prevent radiation upset (2 marks). Some patients experience retrosternal pain when the mediastinum is irradiated, and if so she should be given soft foods (2 marks).

As the treatment lowers the patient's resistance to infection, she should be protected against people with colds and sore throats (2 marks). Mild aperients may be necessary (1 mark).

The skin of the patient's chest wall may become red and sore after 2 or 3 weeks treatment (3 marks). It may even blister (1 mark), or ulcerate, and this will heal slowly (1 mark). Nurses must watch for skin reactions and report them before the skin breaks (1 mark). The area must not be washed (1 mark), and the patient must understand about this; it can be kept dry with baby powder (1 mark). (N.B. as some doctors allow cream to be used, count 1 mark for saying this, instead of powder). Care should be taken not to wash off any skin markings from the radiation field (1 mark). Loose clothing should be worn to prevent friction (1 mark), and skin should not be exposed to excessive heat or cold (1 mark)

When treatment is finished, instructions must be given the patient about care of the skin and when she can start washing the area (1 mark). She should be reassured that the increased pigmentation will not show (1 mark), as it will be hidden by clothes.

During the course of treatment, the patient may feel very unwell (1 mark). Symptoms such as depression and lassitude (1 mark), headache (1 mark), nausea and vomiting (*or* anorexia) (1 mark) are not uncommon. These can be relieved by the administration of pyridoxine (*or* vitamin B_6) (1 mark), chlorpromazine (*or* Largactil) (1 mark) and anti-emetics such as perphenazine (Fentazin) or promethazine (Avomine) (1 for any 1 example). Again the patient should be reassured that the symptoms will pass when treatment is over (2 marks).